Toward the 21st Century

Incorporating Genetics into Primary Health Care

Toward the 21st Century

Incorporating Genetics into Primary Health Care

NANCY TOUCHETTE
Science Designs, Inc.

NEIL A. HOLTZMAN, M.D., M.P.H.
The Johns Hopkins Medical Institutions

JESSICA G. DAVIS, M.D., F.A.C.M.G.
The New York Hospital–Cornell University Medical College

SUZANNE FEETHAM, Ph.D., R.N., F.A.A.N.
University of Illinois at Chicago

Afterword by
FRANCIS S. COLLINS, M.D., Ph.D.
National Human Genome Research Institute

COLD SPRING HARBOR LABORATORY PRESS
1997

ACKNOWLEDGMENT

This publication and the conferences on which it is based were made possible by a grant from The Robert Wood Johnson Foundation.

Cover photo © Billy Barnes/Stock Boston

Library of Congress Cataloging-in-Publications Data

Toward the 21st century : incorporating genetics into primary health
    care / Nancy Touchette ... [et al.].
        p. cm.
    Includes bibliographical references.
    ISBN 0-87969-499-8 (alk. paper)
    1. Medical genetics--Forecasting--Congresses. 2. Primary care
(Medicine)--Forecasting--Congresses. I. Touchette, Nancy.
    [DNLM: 1. Genetics, Medical--trends--congresses. 2. Primary
Health Care--trends--congresses. QZ 50 T737 1997]
RB155.T69 1997
616'.042--dc21
DNLM/DLC
for Library of Congress   97-19247
                                                                    CIP

All Cold Spring Harbor Laboratory Press publications may be ordered directly from Cold Spring Harbor Laboratory Press, 10 Skyline Drive, Plainview, New York 11803-2500. Phone: 1-800-843-4388 in Continental U.S. and Canada. All other locations: (516) 349-1930. FAX: (516) 349-1946. E-mail: cshpress@cshl.org. For a complete catalog of all Cold Spring Harbor Laboratory Press publications, visit our World Wide Web Site http://www.cshl.org/

Contents

Preface

Human genetics was a very difficult field of research for the first three-quarters of this century. The number of human chromosomes was not determined correctly until 1956. The first human disorder caused by a chromosomal abnormality was identified only in 1959, and it was not until 1968 that a gene was assigned to a chromosome other than the X chromosome. Then, in 1972, gene cloning became possible and with the first cloning of a human gene (isolating it in the test tube), a new era began in human genetics. Recombinant DNA techniques have been extraordinarily successful in unraveling the intricacies of human genetic disorders, so much so that the last quarter of the 20th century will be regarded as the golden age of human genetics.

The driving force behind this research is the desire to understand, diagnose, and treat human inherited disorders. As quickly as human disease genes were found and cloned, medical geneticists began to use them for diagnostic purposes. DNA-based techniques, because of their accuracy, reliability, and speed, have become the standard for diagnosis wherever they can be applied.

These tests have benefited many hundreds of families. However, the availability of DNA-based diagnosis creates, or at least exacerbates, many problems in the provision of health care. Questions have arisen, for example, about access to genetic services. What should these services cost and how can they be provided on an equitable basis? What relationship, if any, should there be between the availability of these services and their outcome, and access to health and life insurance? What are the implications of screening populations for genetic disorders? How do we manage the issues of privacy and confidentiality that surround the collection of genetic data? What about the human resources needed: the training and education of genetic counselors and primary care providers such as physicians and nurses?

Genetic analysis has progressed most rapidly with so-called single-gene disorders that afflict small numbers of people. However, we are approaching a time when it will be possible to diagnose genetic predisposition to disorders such as cancers, heart diseases, and mental disorders, which affect millions of individuals. The scale of the current concerns about DNA diagnosis will thus be magnified many-fold. As so often happens, the speed of scientific research is outstripping the development of a reasoned social response to the research.

The scale of response needed may be formidable. It has been argued, for example, that genetic diagnosis will hasten the development of a national health care system in the U.S. by forcing changes in the health insurance industry.

In 1993, Cold Spring Harbor Laboratory approached the Robert Wood Johnson Foundation with a proposal for a series of discussion meetings on the impact of advances in human genetics on health care. The project's objectives were to initiate an examination of health care and related problems arising from the use of human molecular genetics for diagnosis of genetic disorders; to identify particular areas of concern; to recommend actions through which foundations and other institutions could have a significant impact; and to disseminate the discussions and conclusions of these discussions. The Foundation recognized the need to look far into the future and provided funding for two meetings and for the production of this report.

In discussions prior to the meetings, an improvement in the education of health care professionals in genetics was identified as a vital need, since the demand for genetic testing will increase as more tests become available, especially for common disorders, and testing becomes simpler and cheaper. Well-trained professionals will be needed to administer and analyze the tests, and to counsel those affected by the results. The first Robert Wood Johnson Foundation-supported meeting, then, reviewed the current status of genetics in primary health care, and the second looked specifically at how best to incorporate genetics and genetics education into medical and nursing practice.

As is customary at Banbury Center meetings, we endeavored to bring together groups with different perspectives, which, despite their common interests, had not had close interactions with each other, at least in the area of genetics. Participants included geneticists, genetic counselors, primary care physicians, nurses, representatives of professional bodies and patient groups, and health policy experts. This report, by Nancy Touchette, Neil A. Holtzman, Jessica G. Davis, and Suzanne Feetham, synthesizes the discussions and findings of the two meetings. It contains recommendations that demand attention as we move inexorably further into the era of genetically informed medicine.

Jan A. Witkowski, Director
The Banbury Center
Cold Spring Harbor Laboratory

Toward the 21st Century

Incorporating Genetics into Primary Health Care

The First Conference on Genetics and Primary Care: The Role of Geneticists and Genetics Counselors

Widely recognized as one of the most dynamic fields of medicine, medical genetics already has had, and will continue to have, a major impact on the practice of clinical medicine. New genetic advances include the expanded recognition of genetic factors in health and disease, the construction of detailed genetic and physical maps of the human genome, and the development of new techniques for DNA sequencing and information transfer. Gene therapy is now a reality. Carrier testing and population-based screening programs for a variety of genetic problems and one category of birth defects are in place.

It is anticipated that the growing array of biochemical and molecular genetic laboratory assays will enable the number of genetic disorders for which screening and testing are possible to expand. New genetic information will also be utilized to develop innovative therapeutic measures. In turn, new genetic knowledge will provide unprecedented opportunities for individuals to learn about their genetic makeup. Such information is likely to play an increasingly important role as individuals and their health care providers discuss related health issues in order to make decisions about their health, including the adoption of preventive/health promotion strategies.

All of these recent developments indicate that there will be an ever-increasing demand for genetic information and genetic services. To meet these demands, all health care providers and the public will need to be informed about new and emerging developments in the field of medical genetics.

How can we meet this challenge? How can we enhance the genetic knowledge of primary care providers, all health care professionals, and the public? What are the issues? The first Banbury Conference on Genetics and Primary Care provided a forum for representatives of consumer genetic support groups (Alliance), public health (federal, state), genetic and nongenetic health care disciplines, and health care foundations to begin to discuss these issues, to formulate interim principles, and to forge problem-solving strategies.

Members of this working group recognized that just as our understanding of human genetics is increasing, sweeping changes are under way nationwide that will change the way in which health care services are provided. Emphasis will be placed on the provision of community-based, comprehensive, coordinated, and cost-effective health care services. General medical services will be provided by primary care providers. Such practitioners include family physicians, general internists, general pediatricians, general obstetrician-gynecologists, and nurse practitioners. Referrals to subspecialists will be discouraged and curtailed.

This means that the role of the primary health care providers in the provision of direct medical genetic services will increase. It is expected that nongenetic medical personnel will not only order most genetic tests, but will also provide the information about these tests. Nongenetic medical personnel will also be directly involved in the care and management of patients and their families with, or at risk for, genetic disease.

There is uncertainty about the role that genetic health care professionals will play in meeting both inpatient and outpatient genetic service and educational needs. Some large health maintenance organizations (HMOs), such as Kaiser, have medical genetic personnel on staff. The majority of HMOs do not. It appears that unless provision is made to include genetic health care professionals in the diagnostic and treatment loop, the opportunities for genetic education of primary care providers and patients will decline.

Other concerns surfaced. Although there are 2500 certified genetic health care workers, the actual number of individuals engaged in the provision of clinical genetic services is small. Many certified geneticists spend full time in laboratory service and/or research activities. Most practicing medical genetic personnel have some teaching responsibilities. However, their primary educational focus is on medical student and house staff teaching. Postdoctoral fellowship training in genetics is paramount in some centers. Few clinical genetic providers are involved in outreach community-based educational efforts.

There are genuine concerns about meeting the medical genetic educational needs of health care trainees. Impending changes in Medicaid will affect funding for postdoctoral medical genetic education. In addition, the total number of medical residents will be reduced. At the same time, the total number of medical subspecialty residents in all disciplines will be cut. More generalists will be trained by all pediatric, internal medicine and obstetrics/gynecology, and family practice residency programs. As the number of subspecialists declines, the number of primary care providers will increase. As a newly recognized medical subspecialty, medical genetics was not factored into the calculations for the nation's future work force. Therefore, medical genetics will have to fight for a small number of medical training program slots. Few schools of nursing and social work provide postgraduate opportunities for education in genetics. The number of new clinical genetic professionals is also unlikely to increase. Yet there will be an ongoing need to train new leaders and teachers in genetics. Such individuals will be needed to perform research, to provide genetic clinical and laboratory services, and to educate our nation's health care work force. Grants or scholarships for postdoctoral training in medical genetics are in short supply. Support is needed for postdoctoral training in genetics.

Fewer medical genetic personnel would mean less exposure to genetics by house staff, medical students, and allied health professionals, and decreased opportunities for training future generalists about medical genetics. A decrease in the number of skilled medical genetic personnel will limit the exposure of house staff, medical students, generalists, and allied health care professionals to newly emerging genetic information. This, in turn, would have a profound impact on the access of consumers to needed genetic information.

There is also the problem of geographic barriers, which curtail interactions between primary care providers and medical genetic personnel. Most clinical genetic personnel work in tertiary care centers and/or in large community medical centers. Some are in industry or in state health departments. There is maldistribution of genetic health care providers. Some states such as California, Texas, and New York have many medical geneticists. Others, such as New Mexico and Mississippi, have few. Alaska does not have any state-based clinical genetic providers.

New strategies to utilize the media for genetic education are required. New educational tools such as interactive computer-based programs need to be developed to encourage home-based study. Telecommunication could be used to facilitate needed interactions between the primary care providers and their back-up regional clinical genetics personnel.

Why are these issues of concern? There are few studies concerning the genetic knowledge of primary health care providers. Such studies reveal a paucity of knowledge about genetic principles, technologies, genetic tests and genetic disease, and susceptibility to disease among primary care providers, medical subspecialists, nurses, social workers, and hospital and managed care administrators.

At the first Banbury Conference, we discussed some existing genetic educational models and learned about several genetic educational programs designed for primary care providers. We focused on successful ingredients for such programs and also learned about the problems. For example, in order to mount a successful educational program, geneticists must survey their target audience about their needs and priorities and not assume that their choice of topics will be of importance to primary care providers. Consumer input would also enhance all such educational efforts. It was clear that geneticists also needed to become more informed about primary care.

Conference participants learned about some new projects. Sponsored by the Genetic Services Branch, Maternal and Child Health Bureau (MCHB), pilot projects are now under way to expand opportunities for genetic education among a variety of primary health care providers. A major goal of these projects is to develop working partnerships between community-based primary care providers and local medical genetic personnel in an effort to pinpoint needs in order to design and develop cooperative educational programs that can be implemented and field tested within a variety of community-based settings. Some of the projects design innovative medical genetic curricula including telecommunication programs. All of these peer-reviewed projects include a rigorous evaluation component. For example, one program is assessing the impact of its educational efforts on its participants' practice parameters and the enhancement of the working relationships between the community-based practitioners and their local genetic service providers.

All of these projects will be subject to in-depth review and on-going monitoring. If successful, these programs could be replicated with appropriate modifications in order to reach large numbers of primary care providers within each of the ten funded regional genetic service networks. It is hoped that these programs will provide needed data on how to make genetic information more accessible, relevant, and user-friendly.

In addition, we exchanged information on a variety of projects sponsored by the Human Genome Project and the national professional genetic and nongenetic organizations to provide genetic education to health care providers and the general public. Data from such programs should also prove helpful in planning future activities.

Since all medical and nursing students will utilize genetic information in the 21st century, questions were raised about the type of genetic instruction currently offered in our nation's medical and nursing schools. Most medical schools offer courses in genetics. Most nursing school curricula offer modules on basic pathogenetic mechanisms. Pertinent information on genetics is incorporated into pediatric and obstetric-gynecology courses. A recent report by the American Society of Human Genetics (ASHG) on a Medical School Core Curriculum was published in 1995 (Friedman, J.M. et al. 1995. ASHG Report. Report from the ASHG Information and Education Committee: Medical School Core Curriculum in Genetics. *Am. J. Hum. Genet.* **199**: **56**: 535–537). It has been well received.

Following the Banbury Conferences, ASHG and the American College of Medical Genetics began to work to increase the number of questions concerning genetics on the national medical board examinations. If successful, this will enable the deans of the nation's medical schools to evaluate the impact of genetic education on their medical students.

The Human Genome Project has funded several highly successful human genetic education projects targeted at high school biology teachers and high school students. Conferees speculated that such projects could be modified to reach larger and broader audiences in order to increase the general population's genetic knowledge.

The first Banbury Conference on Genetics and Primary Care served as a catalyst. Participants were able to review what has been accomplished as well as to understand the problems. By focusing on the genetic educational needs in primary care, the group realized that much work must be done before the genetic work load escalates due to increased screening for susceptibility to common diseases. Primary care providers will play a major role in informing patients about the array of genetic services and assays, acting as patient advocates, making appropriate referrals, and working closely with the medical genetic community.

Much can and will be achieved through long-range planning and cooperative professionally led initiatives. Medical genetics is not the sole responsibility of the medical genetic community, because its effects will be increasingly felt throughout all of medicine and society. In order for medical genetics to be fully incorporated into the mainstream of medicine, it is essential that all health care practitioners be fully informed about its power and relevance.

Jessica G. Davis

The Second Conference on Genetics and Primary Care: The Role of Primary Care Providers and Medical Educators

In the year after the second Banbury Conference on genetics and primary care, two gene loci have been discovered at which inherited mutations increase susceptibility to breast cancer. Several clinical laboratories began to offer testing for these mutations to asymptomatic persons. In addition, evidence accumulated that a common genetic variant, apolipoprotein e4, is a risk factor for Alzheimer's disease. Some predictive testing was done for this protein. Scientists also reported gene loci at which inherited mutations increase the risk of diabetes mellitus, schizophrenia, and bipolar affective disorder. As Francis Collins pointed out in his keynote address to the second meeting (see elsewhere in this volume), the genome project was, and remains, ahead of schedule, accelerating discoveries like those described.

Collins also pointed out that "(t)he mass media are currently the major carrier of information about genetic medicine to the public. Some of the information is accurate and some of it isn't—but more and more, patients are bringing the magazine or the newspaper into the health care provider's office wanting to know if they are genetically prone to a given disease." Unless physicians know how to answer these queries, and unless they know what tests to detect "proneness" are available and when they are indicated, patients will not be well served. At the first Banbury conference, the emphasis was on programs created by geneticists to educate health care providers about genetics and genetic services outreach programs. Participants at the second conference explored the needs and perceptions of primary care providers, including those involved in managed care, and considered how genetics could be better integrated into medical and nursing education. As a prelude to the second conference, we elicited the attitudes of invitees (including a few who declined to attend) about the types of genetic services that are most important for primary care and about the greatest needs of primary care practitioners (see elsewhere in this volume).

Why do genetic services warrant so much concern? One reason is that the discovery of disease-related genes enables us to identify people who have inherited mutations that increase their risk of future disease before we have the ability to prevent or ameliorate the disease. As Collins points out, this "time lag...has raised questions about whether we are really ready to offer testing." Yet academic and commercial clinical laboratories make tests available, and reporting in the mass media often implies that the information is something that people want or should have. Not only are few treatments available, but also, as Collins points out, genetic information can lead to loss of insurance and employment. Moreover, the information itself may be inaccurate, presenting another reason for concern.

The most straightforward interpretation of a positive genetic test result can be made for the relatively rare diseases (cystic fibrosis, sickle cell anemia, thalassemia, and Tay-Sachs are among the most frequent of them) whose inheritance follows the rules first observed by Gregor Mendel. Paradoxically, however, it is tests for common complex disorders, such as cancer and Alzheimer's disease, that receive the most attention, including commercial test development. A positive result for these disorders by no means guarantees that the person will develop the disorder. Five to ten percent of people with breast or colon cancer inherit mutations that greatly increase their susceptibility to developing cancer, but they must *acquire* mutations in the homologous gene and in other independently inherited genes before malignant transformation occurs. The likelihood of these additional mutations is affected by exposure to mutagens and other factors still unknown. For one form of colon cancer (familial adenomatous polyposis [FAP]) the likelihood of these secondary changes is extremely high, probably more than 95%, but for other forms of familial colon cancer and for the familial forms of breast cancer, the chance, although still high, is less than 85%. These risk estimates are derived from "cancer families" in which at least two first-degree relatives have cancer. When inherited susceptibility mutations (ISMs) are found in healthy people without a family history of cancer, the chance that cancer will develop could be much lower. They are less likely than members of cancer families to share alleles at other gene loci that increase sensitivity to environmental factors, or to share exposure to such factors. The average chance of getting Alzheimer's disease if one has a family history and possesses a single apolipoprotein e4 allele is only about 50% and is lower in men than in women and in some ethnic groups than in others, again suggesting the influence of other factors, probably environmental and genetic.

For common, complex disorders like diabetes or schizophrenia, there is little evidence that susceptibility is greatly increased by the presence of ISMs at a single gene locus. Instead, the simultaneous presence of ISMs at several loci, along with environmental factors, is needed. Even if scientists were to discover all of the gene loci at which ISMs contributed to the occurrence of these diseases, the yield would be low. For instance, if the simultaneous presence of ISMs at three independently segregating gene loci accounts for some patients with schizophrenia, and the frequency of ISMs at each of these loci is 1%, then the chance that a person in the general population would possess ISMs at all three loci is 0.01^3, or 1 in 1 million, orders of magnitude lower than the frequency of schizophrenia.

The difficulty of interpreting positive test results in healthy people hinges on disease etiology and pathogenesis, not on technology. This is only partly true for negative results. We now know that multiple disease-related mutations exist at many gene loci, over 600 at the cystic fibrosis gene locus and over 100 at the BRCA1 locus, and still counting. Short of sequencing the entire gene, which is extremely expensive and time-consuming, these mutations cannot all be detected. Thus, with one important exception, people with negative test results cannot be reassured that they will remain free of the disease; they may possess an undetectable mutation, or the disease could result from other factors. The exception arises in families in which affected relatives possess an inherited mutation that is known to have played a major role in their contracting the disease. Finding that the mutation is absent in a relative at risk reduces the chance of disease toward the chance in the general population. For a Mendelian condition like Huntington's disease, this would be close to zero. For inherited susceptibility to breast cancer, finding that a healthy woman does not possess the BRCA1 ISM found in her affected relatives reduces her chance of contracting breast cancer from approximately 85% to 12%. A number of new technologies offer promise of improving the detection rate of ISMs, but these are years off.

Another reason for concern about genetic tests is the information they convey about risks to children. Although the principal reason to test for ISMs for adult-onset disease is to reduce the chance of disease in the people being tested, the finding of an ISM in a parent immediately indicates that his or her children have a 50% chance of also having it. Parents might want this information even if nothing could be done to reduce the risk of future disease in their children. Occasionally, as in FAP and a few other disorders, the discovery that an ISM is absent saves the child from undergoing invasive monitoring procedures to look for early signs of disease. For most adult-onset diseases, however, the first evidence does not appear until adulthood, and there is no need for monitoring minors or undertaking prophylactic measures.

Prospective parents with an ISM might want to avoid having a child with an ISM. One way of doing this is to use prenatal diagnosis and to terminate the pregnancy if an ISM is found. This raises thorny ethical questions of whether termination is justified when the disease in question will not appear until adulthood and when an effective intervention might be found before it does appear. So far, few parents seem interested in prenatal diagnosis for adult-onset disorders, but the fact that it's an option raises the difficult question of how information should be conveyed to adults considering testing for the chance of future disease in themselves.

This brings us to a final reason for concern: the way information is communicated to users of genetic services. Until now, most genetic counseling has been provided by medical geneticists and genetic counselors to parents concerned about their chances of having children with a specific disease. To avoid the taint of eugenics, these professionals attempt to give information in a nondirective manner, permitting counselees to make autonomous decisions consonant with their own values. As Nancy Touchette describes elsewhere in this volume, our group has found that primary care providers are less likely than genetic professionals to be nondirective when dealing with reproductive options. In testing for adult-onset diseases, however, the major reason for testing will be reducing the chance of disease in the person being tested. If disease is highly likely in those with positive test results, and highly unlikely in those with negative results, and if safe, effective interventions can prevent or ameliorate disease, perhaps providers should recommend the test. As we have seen, this ideal situation is seldom attained today. Considerable uncertainty surrounds both positive and negative results in tests for ISMs, and few safe and effective therapies have been discovered. There are, moreover, the reproductive implications when ISMs are detected. For all these reasons, a nondirective approach seems appropriate. Although we have found that consumers often want a recommendation from their provider about having a genetic test, they want to hear all of the options and make the final decision themselves.

Primary care and other nongenetic providers might conclude from this discussion that there is little chance that they will have to confront genetic testing. They may ask, If the tests are so imperfect and of questionable utility, how will they get into practice? Currently, no regulatory authority except New York State examines whether genetic tests offered by clinical laboratories have been scientifically validated and have clinical utility. Although both academic and commercial laboratories offering genetic tests must register with the Health Care Financing Administration (HCFA) under the Clinical Laboratory Improvement Amendments, HCFA has no authority to look at scientific validation and clinical utility. The Task Force on Genetic Testing, which I chair, is looking into policies for changing this situation.

Nongenetic providers might also assume that they can simply refer patients to medical geneticists and genetic counselors. There are only about 2000 genetic professionals in the United States, and their number is not increasing. They can handle the demand for counseling families at high risk for single-gene diseases and many ISMs, but if tests are marketed to the general population, they are far too few to provide initial education and counseling to all those who might be interested. Managed care organizations, moreover, may be unwilling to permit many referrals. Given the long time it takes to counsel patients, and the fast pace of primary care practice, new approaches to providing information and counseling must be found. Training nurses to fulfill genetics education and counseling roles received considerable attention at the second conference. In developing new modalities, the viewpoints and preferences of consumers need to be considered. They should be involved in planning new services.

Primary care providers will have to confront the issues raised by genetic testing. In the sections that follow, many approaches to the issues that must be resolved are considered. We have the opportunity of finding solutions before the problem gets out of hand.

The Banbury conferences on primary care have already had at least three salutary effects. First, all 28 of the participants at the second conference who responded to a brief questionnaire several months after the conference (85% of those attending) said they discussed the meeting with their colleagues, Of these, 23 said they planned further activities related to the conference topics. One area in which intensive follow-up has already occurred is nursing education. Second, the Robert Wood Johnson Foundation agreed to a request of participants at the second conference to support a study of the extent to which genetic services are being incorporated into managed care and how this is being accomplished. Third, Genetic Services Branch of the Maternal and Child Health Bureau, USDHSS, is undertaking a parallel study of efforts to educate primary care providers about genetics.

Neil A. Holtzman

Integrating Genetics into Primary Health Care

Prologue

The 1990s might be considered the decade in which the science of genetics came into its own. The discovery of new ways to manipulate DNA has led to a remarkable revolution in genetics. Genetic research has reached a dizzying pace as researchers appear to unearth new genes almost daily. Understanding how mutations in specific genes contribute to diseases such as neurofibromatosis, cancer, cystic fibrosis, and muscular dystrophy may ultimately improve treatment. Although instant cures are not expected, researchers believe that the discovery of the genetic mutations that affect risk for disease may help patients to plan their course of treatment, make decisions about their reproductive future, and make adjustments in life-style and behavior.

If the 1990s can be heralded as the decade of gene discovery, the challenge as we head toward the turn of the century and beyond is to incorporate some of the newly acquired knowledge in medical genetics into mainstream health care. Already many recent genetic advances have given rise to new diagnostic tools; but if there is to be a widespread application of genetic testing in diagnosing and ultimately treating diseases with genetic components, will the health care system be prepared to deal with the new advances? Who will provide consumers with the information and counseling they will need to make informed decisions about their well-being?

The Banbury Center, under the sponsorship of the Robert Wood Johnson Foundation, hosted two workshops to assess the extent to which the current health care system is ready to meet the challenge of the revolution in human genetics. The first Banbury Center meeting on Human Genetics and Health Care, held August 28–31, 1994, enabled clinical geneticists and genetic counselors to outline the issues involved in the delivery of genetic services. The meeting, organized by Dale Lea, a registered nurse and genetic counselor at the Foundation for Blood Research in Scarborough, Maine, and Jessica Davis, a medical geneticist at Cornell University College of Medicine, was attended in large part by geneticists and genetic counselors, with a smattering of nurses, primary care physicians, and public health and social service professionals. Geneticists acknowledged that they could not meet the future demand for genetic services and that many routine services will increasingly fall on the shoulders of primary care practitioners. Discussions centered on what primary care practitioners ought to know about genetics to meet the anticipated demand for genetic services in the coming years. A second meeting, Incorporating Genetics into Medicine and Nursing Education and Practice, also sponsored by the Robert Wood Johnson Foundation, was held at the Banbury Center April 1–3, 1995.

"At the first meeting, we focused on the appropriate services to be delivered," said Neil Holtzman, a medical geneticist from Johns Hopkins University. "But it was not clear that what we want reflects reality. We didn't know how receptive primary care providers would be to this fledgling discipline." Meeting participants developed a list of recommended goals, which are summed on pages 44–46 and 59–60.

The focus of the second meeting, attended by a large percentage of nurses and physicians in primary care, was on the needs of primary care providers: What do they want or need to know to deliver genetic services to their patients? Participants targeted two main areas of concern: incorporating genetics into primary care practice and introducing genetics into medical and nursing education.

"The goal is to find a realistic approach as we ask ourselves, Are we ready to incorporate genetics into health disciplines?" said Holtzman. "Is there a need and can we fulfill it to ensure that the public receives services safely and effectively?" A second goal, said Holtzman, is to develop "very concrete plans to incorporate genetics into medicine and nursing. We would like to come up with specific models to accomplish this."

The meetings were significant in that they relied heavily on the input from the very people who will ultimately carry genetics to the vast majority of people seeking services: the primary care practitioners. Clearly, geneticists, genetic counselors, nurses, and doctors all have differing perspectives on how best to deliver such services, and the meetings brought out some of those differences. The meetings also served an important function by identifying the commonalities and bringing together people with complementary talents to begin to think about how best to proceed with the enormous task of integrating genetics into mainstream medicine. Although the task is far from over, meeting organizers and participants have taken an important first step toward laying the groundwork to ultimately move genetics and the care of persons into 21st-century medicine.

At the Outset

The ultimate goal of medical research is to improve the health of the general populace. Although genetic advances may not produce any magic bullets for curing disease, many researchers and health care professionals point out that genetic testing and services have already had an effect on health care, and that influence is expected to increase in the years to come.

"Will it change our understanding of the etiology, our approach to, and the prevention of disease?" asks Philip Reilly, a physician and medical geneticist at the Shriver Center for Mental Retardation in Waltham, Massachusetts. "How can we maximize the use of genetic testing and minimize the potential harm introduced by the new knowledge?" At the first Banbury meeting, Reilly posed several central questions worth addressing as geneticists, primary care practitioners, and policymakers consider the future of genetic testing and the delivery of genetic services:

- Is it possible to engage in central planning about how new genetic technologies should flow into the clinical sector?

- To what extent are patterns of genetic service delivery really altered by pressures from the commercial sector?

- What will be the influence of malpractice litigation on the pace at which new tests and services are brought on line?

- To what extent will reimbursement constraints affect the orderly evolution of services (who will pay?)

- What is the adequate core knowledge base in genetics for the primary care practitioner?

- What is the adequate knowledge base for nurses, physicians, social workers, and other medical specialists who will work in genetics?

- How do we convince medical and nursing educators to believe in the need for more genetics knowledge and to find more room in curricula for genetics?

- Is a massive effort at consumer education a realistic goal?

- Is it possible to project the actual demand curve for genetic services 5 or 10 years hence?

- Are we making much ado about very little? That is, if we do nothing special will genetic services trickle into health care much the way as other technologies?

Throughout the course of the first Banbury meeting, participants addressed many of Reilly's questions, sometimes arriving at answers, but more often than not, inviting further questions. However, the meeting served as an important first step in defining some of the key issues that must be dealt with if genetics is to move successfully into mainstream health care.

State of Genetic Services

What Are Genetic Services?

Genetic services consist of much more than simply disclosing the results of genetic tests. Genetic services can include the assessment and diagnosis of medical conditions with genetic components, genetic testing, and genetic counseling. Genetic counseling is a communication process that deals with the human problems associated with a genetic disorder or the risk of a genetic disorder occurring within a family (NIH and National Genetics Foundation, adopted by the American Society of Human Genetics, 1975). Through genetic counseling, trained professionals try to help affected individuals and families to

- understand the medical information available, including the probable course of the disorder, and treatment and management options available

- appreciate the contribution of heredity to the disorder and the risk of occurrence in other family members

- understand the options for dealing with the risk of recurrence and choose the course of action that seems appropriate to them in view of their risk and the family goals

- act in accordance with any decisions made by the client

- make the best possible adjustment to the disorder

Because many individuals and families seek genetic counseling—either before conception or during pregnancy—to determine whether future family members might be affected, it is important that patients understand the options available for dealing with the risk of occurrence of the disease in future family members. These options might include artificial insemination, surrogacy, adoption, foster parenting, prenatal testing, elective pregnancy termination, and birth control. Genetic counseling can also help individuals at risk for adult-onset diseases develop coping strategies and treatment options.

Once a patient has chosen a particular course of action, genetic counselors also attempt to help him or her adjust to the genetic condition by discussing coping strategies, exploring goals and expectations, and integrating family and cultural values and religious beliefs. Counselors may also make referrals when appropriate and provide continued support.

Who Seeks Genetic Counseling?

Although people may seek genetic services for many different reasons, the vast majority do so because they have had a child with a genetic disease or a genetic disorder. "Usually, people ask, Why did it happen? Will it happen again? What can I do about it?" says Ann Walker, a genetic counselor at the

University of California at Irvine. "They want to know if they are at fault." The following are typical situations. A couple has just given birth to a child with phenylketonuria and wants to know what caused the disorder and whether it will happen again. A 37-year-old woman is pregnant and wants to know the chances of having a child with Down's syndrome. A couple with a history of miscarriages or birth defects wants to know the likelihood of carrying a healthy child to term. A pregnant woman has been exposed to radiation and wants to know whether it will affect her baby. Some clients want to know what the risks are before they conceive a child.

Frequently, clients seek genetic services if there is a family history of an inherited disease that occurs later in life. A woman with a mother and sister who died of breast cancer may want to know what her chances are of developing the disease and what she can do to prevent it. Relatives of a family member affected by Huntington's disease may want to know if they will meet the same fate.

Often, clients seek genetic services for diagnosis. A child may develop cafe-au-lait spots, and geneticists may be called upon to help determine the cause. A 15-year-old who has not yet gone through puberty may seek the services of a medical geneticist to figure out why. There are many tests to help physicians and genetic counselors diagnose genetic conditions and determine whether individuals carry altered genes that may lead to disease. For example, currently, newborns are tested for a variety of metabolic conditions, including sickle cell anemia, phenylketonuria, and hypothyroidism; adults can be tested for susceptibility to certain cancers; and amniocentesis can determine whether a fetus will be affected by Down's syndrome, cystic fibrosis, neural tube defects, or Tay-Sachs disease. Adults can also be tested to see if they are carriers for recessive diseases such as sickle cell anemia and thalassemia.

Except for prenatal diagnosis and many predictive tests for single-gene disorders, medical genetics is still a science of uncertainty. Genetics professionals can examine a family tree, run a battery of tests, and evaluate various life-style factors, but at best they can only tell their clients the probability of developing or inheriting a particular condition. Mystery still abounds: Assessing risk for genetics disorders, for the most part, remains largely speculative. The revolution in genetics will undoubtedly lead to the availability of more tools to allow physicians to predict the probability of and to diagnose genetic disease with more certainty. However, the need for genetic services will likely increase exponentially as more tests become available. Patients—even those whose tests bear good news—need to understand the full implications of testing and how it will affect their lives and those of their offspring and other relatives. They do not need to have decisions made for them, but rather to be provided with enough correct information to make their own decisions.

Members of the health care community agree that the present level of genetic services will not be sufficient to meet the rising demand for such services as genetic information becomes increasingly available. Many physicians, nurses, genetic counselors, and medical geneticists feel that action must be taken now to meet the demands of the present and future.

What Are the Goals of Providing Genetic Services?

As more people are trained to provide genetic services, many consider it crucial that goals, philosophy, and ethical standards of genetic service providers are not compromised. Ann Walker, speaking at the first Banbury meeting, emphasized that the manner in which genetic services are dispensed is as important as the factual information provided. "Genetic counseling is traditionally delivered in a nondirective way," said Walker. "We don't tell patients what they should do. The purpose is non-eugenic. It's not a way to improve the gene pool. There is a need to be respectful of patient autonomy."

Walker and other speakers also emphasized that fully informed consent is an issue in genetic counseling. Before agreeing to counseling, patients need to be aware of the aspects of psychological harm that may be introduced by genetic counseling. For example, in a family affected by a fatal adult-onset disease, for which there is no cure, do patients really want to know their fate?

Confidentiality is also paramount. The issue of what types of genetic information, if any, insurance agencies, employers, and others should have access to remains the subject of intense debate. In lieu of legislation to protect the privacy of patients, they need assurance that any information disclosed during genetic counseling will remain confidential.

Walker says it is also important that genetic counseling be tailored to the needs and educational level of clients. In addition, genetic information and counseling must be sensitive to the cultural needs of the community.

Who Provides Genetic Services?

Fewer than 1000 physicians in the United States today are trained to provide genetic information to their patients. Only 200 nurses identify themselves as providers of genetic information, and there are currently fewer than 1000 genetic counselors. All told, fewer than 2500 professionals identify themselves as providers of genetic information. However, not all medical genetics professionals see patients and/or counsel them. "Most genetic counseling is conducted in academic medical centers and is strongly linked to research," says Philip Reilly.

Over the past decade, there has been a shift in the delivery of genetic services. For example, in 1981, 59% of all genetic services were provided by university medical centers and 19% by large community-based medical centers. In 1992, 51% of all genetic services were delivered in academic (university) settings, and 28% of services were provided by medical centers. During the same period, services provided by private hospitals increased from 19% to 28% and that of HMOs from 0.7% to 5.5%, while services by outreach and government public health clinics dropped (see Table 1).

Although their numbers are small, medical geneticists and genetic counselors provide the bulk of genetic services to consumers today. As the need increases, however, and as the delivery of services shifts from academic centers to private hospitals, managed care, and HMOs, other health care professionals may be called upon to provide genetic counseling. Nurses, primary health care physicians, obstetricians, pediatricians, internists, medical specialists, and social workers who are already providing some genetic services may be recruited as future genetic service providers.

MEDICAL GENETICISTS

Medical geneticists are usually clinicians holding an M.D. or Ph.D. Among physicians, medical geneticists come from several different medical disciplines, with a large number involved with children and pediatric diseases. Of physicians certified by the American College of Human Genetics, 60% are pediatricians, 11% are obstetrician/gynecologists, 12% are internists, and 17% come from other fields (e.g., pathology, general practice, neurology).

According to Jessica Davis, medical geneticists are usually trained at the postdoctoral level. Physicians can train as medical geneticists by completing an approved fellowship program in medical genetics, following residency. This may involve 2 years of clinical training, culminating with the presentation of a clinical project, and followed by a third year of laboratory science. Candidates can also complete a residency program in genetics following graduation from medical school.

There are, however, barriers looming that threaten delivery of genetic services by medical geneticists in the future. Anticipated changes in the United States funding of postdoctoral education may present a major obstacle to those present and future health care professionals who desire to provide genetic services. Additional problems arise from the inequitable geographic distribution of trained clinical geneticists. Although the largest numbers of geneticists are located in California and New York, some states have only a

Table 1. Distribution of Genetic Services

Location of service or counselors	1981	1992
University/medical center	59%	51%
Federal/state/county office	8%	4%
Outreach	4.7%	1.3%
Private hospital	19.3%	27.6%
HMO	0.7%	5.5%

Table from Ann Walker (pers. comm.). Data from National Society of Genetic Counselors.

few and others lack clinical geneticists entirely. New Mexico, for example, has only three medical geneticists and Alaska has none. Each of these issues presents a different challenge to be overcome by the health care community in the promotion of genetic services as a component of primary care.

GENETIC COUNSELORS

Approximately 1000 genetic counselors holding M.S. degrees currently practice in the United States. Membership in the National Society of Genetic Counselors has risen to 934 members, 814 of whom are board-certified to practice genetic counseling. Most genetic counselors (87%) practice in a clinical setting, usually at an academic medical center or private hospital. Of genetic counselors, 57% conduct prenatal counseling and some are involved in screening programs in public health settings.

In 1994, only 105 master's level genetic counselors graduated in the United States. Currently, only 17 universities offer genetic counseling programs. Clinical training throughout the country varies widely. Graduates of some programs spend only 400 hours in the clinic, whereas other programs require more than 2000 hours of clinical training. Although the average cost of earning a masters degree in genetic counseling is approximately $8,000, the costs vary widely, ranging from $1,900 to $16,000. Training fellowships to support genetic counseling trainees are virtually nonexistent.

"Why can't we train more?" asked Walker at the Banbury meeting. "The University of California at Irvine only admits 4 out of nearly 100 candidates each year. There are only 100 slots for approximately 600 candidates nationwide each year." Part of the problem, says Walker, is that genetic counseling is not a lucrative business. "Universities don't see genetic counselors as a source for producing research money. We don't have the financial support to expand our programs."

NURSES

Although the nursing profession does not offer certification in genetics, nurses with training in genetics have been drawn into the field of genetic service in increasing capacities over the past several decades. According to Janet Williams, a nurse at the University of Iowa in Iowa City, in the 1960s many nurses identified individuals at risk for genetic disorders in the community and counseled them, a role which continues. Throughout the 1970s, nurses, as genetic counseling team members, became involved in maternal and child health and expanded their involvement in risk identification and counseling. Clinical nurses specializing in genetics began to appear in the 1980s, as they became involved in direct care of patients with genetic disease, the education of professionals, consultation, and research. The focus for the 1990s, says Williams, is research into coping mechanisms and concerns with prenatal screening and understanding the nature of genetic conditions. "Increasingly, we are seeing the incorporation of genetic principles into nursing practice—in school nursing, critical care nursing, oncology, cardiology, primary care, and public health," says Williams.

Indeed, the more than 2 million registered nurses practicing in the United States today may serve as a tremendous untapped resource to deliver genetic services in the future (see pages 42–43.) However, the widespread use of nurses as providers of genetic services may require drastic changes in nursing curricula. According to a 1994 survey of nurses conducted by the American Nurses Association, only 9% of all nurses had ever taken a course in genetics (see pages 49–52.) A 1984 survey of nursing instructors demonstrated that most schools provide less than 10 hours of instruction in genetics (Forsman 1988).

Do Consumers Want Expanded Access to Genetic Services?

Implicit throughout most discussions calling for an increase in the number of geneticists and genetic counselors is the assumption that there is indeed a need or demand for such services. New genes and genetic mutations that lead to disease are being discovered rapidly and the availability of genetic tests is increasing exponentially. But who wants the tests? Consumers? The physicians? Corporations marketing the tests?

For many diseases, the availability of genetic tests may create as many problems as it purports to remedy. The dilemma is especially acute for diseases such as Huntington's disease or cystic fibrosis, for which there is no cure. If the available options upon discovering that one carries a gene for a genetic disorder included a successful prevention, treatment, or cure, patients at high risk might be flocking to test centers. But for many diseases, this is not the case.

Katherine Schneider, a genetic counselor at the Dana Farber Cancer Institute, studies the genetics of cancer. She has counseled members of families at high risk for Li-Fraumeni syndrome—a rare inherited cancer syndrome—and family members who have a high risk of breast cancer. Schneider and her colleagues offered members of these families genetic counseling and testing for genes that are known to be associated with the inherited cancers (see section on Service Models, p. 27). Among families affected by Li-Fraumeni syndrome, none wanted genetic testing to determine whether they would develop the syndrome. Among 200 members of a family with a history of breast cancer, only 1 accepted an offer of genetic counseling, and 2 expressed an interest in testing and counseling.

"We find that similar to Huntington's disease, 95% of clients in families at risk for cancer don't want testing," said Schneider at the first Banbury meeting. "It's difficult to find a time when they can cope, while they are already dealing with losses in their families." According to Schneider, one patient had a dying brother, another was going through the process of bone marrow donation, and another was coping with the recent deaths of a cousin and father. "There's no good time to be tested," says Schneider. "In AIDS testing, there is a similar scenario. Some individuals test, but they often don't come back for their results. Although some patients will opt for vigorous screening, others don't want to think about it."

Schneider says that each individual has his or her own reasons for being tested for adult-onset diseases such as cancer, and much depends on the patient's perception of whether or not the information will help in treating or preventing disease. In her recent book *Counseling About Cancer: Strategies for Genetic Counselors*, she quotes two different patients from families at high risk for cancer and their reasons for seeking or not seeking genetic testing for a predisposition to Li-Fraumeni syndrome:

> I have had cancer three times...and at present time I am the only surviving member of my family who has had cancer. In knowing a member of a family carries the altered gene, I believe a person can make informed choices about lifestyle and career choices and also be aware of changes that may lead to an early detection of cancer. I know I would have my three daughters tested. My sister also wants to be tested. Although she is in her 30s and has never had cancer, she worries every time any problem arises that it may be caused by cancer.

> I have twice been diagnosed with cancer...[and] when I was first diagnosed, it was pain-fully obvious that I had inherited this disease. Our family pedigree spoke for itself. I now have a [young] daughter, and, in spite of our history, I will not have her tested for the gene. I see more problems from knowing than good. Who can predict which of us is capable of handling the news of this altered gene? We all know with certainty that we are at high risk of cancer and should be vigilant about our health...as I see it, testing does little more than end the uncertainty of genetic cancer. For me, it seems right to accept the hand that is dealt, cherish each day with my family and continue to pray for our good health and a cure.

Many participants of the Banbury meeting expressed uncertainty over whether the demand for genetic testing will indeed increase as more genetic tests become available. "Virtually nothing has been published on the projected demand for genetic testing and genetic services," says Philip Reilly. "I don't know that we have the data and I don't know that we can develop it. But I think it's probably going to increase and it's going to be driven by malpractice lawsuits."

Neil Holtzman, a geneticist at Johns Hopkins University, has studied the factors associated with a patient's willingness to undergo testing for mutations in the cystic fibrosis gene. In 1994, he and his colleagues reported (*Am. J. Hum. Gen.* **55**: 626–637 [1994]) that convenience may be as important as philosophical preferences in deciding whether or not to undergo testing. Holtzman and his coworkers invited non-pregnant patients with no family history of cystic fibrosis to test for whether they might carry mutant, disease-associated forms of the gene. To develop cystic fibrosis, a person must inherit two altered, or mutant, copies of the CFTR gene. If a person inherits one mutated CFTR gene and one normal gene, he or she will not develop cystic fibrosis but can pass it on to offspring. Such individuals, known as carriers, may thus be capable of giving birth to children with cystic fibrosis even if they do not have the disease themselves.

The researchers found that when they mailed invitations to patients offering a test for CF carrier status, only 3.7% followed through by responding to a questionnaire, attending a group educational session, and ultimately, deciding to have the test. In contrast, when individuals were approached in an HMO and offered the test on the spot, 23.5% submitted to the test.

Among the reasons patients cited as factors in being tested were convenience and cost, and the desire or possibility of having children in the future. Other studies have also shown that although the interest in having a test for CF carrier status is relatively high even in non-pregnant populations, the utilization is low, particularly when having the test requires an expenditure of time and/or money. The desire for convenience on the part of the public may be at odds with the concerns of geneticists and genetic counselors who feel that it is important that those receiving genetic tests be adequately counseled.

"The marketing of tests commercially available is at variance with genetic counselors, who tend to take a much more conservative approach," said George Cunningham of the California Department of Health Services in Berkeley. "The genetics community often publishes very conservative statements cautioning that a particular commercial test may not be ready for general application." Cunningham says that genetic counselors and medical geneticists are much more likely to approve of newly marketed genetic tests only under certain conditions. In addition, says Cunningham, geneticists want assurance that once tested, patients will have adequate access to counseling services.

"You also have to demonstrate that we have a system that not only deals with intent but also attends to the consequences of [genetic] testing," says Cunningham. "Are there enough CF centers to refer patients to? Do we have enough trained counselors to counsel patients?"

Some conference participants also voiced a further concern that the desire for genetic testing may arise not from the patients themselves, but from personal motives among medical professionals and in private industry. "The issue of demand is a malleable concept," said Elizabeth Thomson, of the Ethical, Legal, and Social Issues (ELSI) program of the National Center for Human Genome Research at the National Institutes of Health in Bethesda. "Sometimes the demand is created by the health care provider."

A patient's desire or willingness to be tested may be affected either by a provider's enthusiasm for testing or by marketing strategies by testing companies. "We have found that we can influence the desire for CF screening," says Holtzman. "It's a matter of marketing—dramatizing the benefits and minimizing the risks. Should we leave this to the private sector?"

In some cases, a patient may be unduly persuaded by a physician to submit to genetic testing when the desire is not present to begin with. "There is a fine line between increasing access and selling services," says Ann Walker. "In a tertiary care center, clients have made a decision to seek genetic services. In a primary care setting, this is not necessarily the case."

In other situations, consumers may be led to genetic testing through newspaper reports and consumer-directed advertisements. Recently, many pharmaceutical companies have taken to advertising for prescription drugs in magazines, newspapers, or on television. "There is a treatment for the flu—you don't have to suffer," the ads purport. "See your doctor today."

"Large pharmaceutical companies produce ads that now directly target patients," says James Allen of the American Medical Association. "There will be pressure on physicians by consumers to have a certain test done. I predict high use of genetic services. We're looking at hundreds of thousands of people potentially interested in tests for breast cancer and colon cancer."

Cunningham voiced skepticism over whether such a scenario would be likely to occur. "I have not yet seen any ground swell of doctors under pressure from malpractice to screen all their patients for colon cancer simply because the newspaper publishes a story about a breakthrough," he said.

Some conference participants believe that patients should have access to information and testing for any genetic tests that become available. "Some will want to be screened for BRCA1 [breast cancer gene], some will not," says Joseph Shulman, of the Genetics and IVF Institute in Fairfax, Virginia, a private laboratory. "What's wrong with that? We need to respect the intelligence of patients."

The role of patient autonomy and self-determination is an actively debated issue of concern to geneticists and patients alike. Often physicians and other health care professionals believe that they are acting in the best interest of the patient even if the patient disagrees. "Genetics is akin to missionaryism," said Kathy Ales, a physician based in Princeton, New Jersey. "You're trying to convince people this is good for you."

Physicians may often believe not only that they are acting in the best interest of the patient, but also that they know what their patients want. To test that notion, Holtzman and his colleagues conducted independent surveys of physicians and consumers to determine what types of genetic information and services the patients were most interested in. The researchers asked a sampling of adults both with and without a family history of CF to rank selected questions in the order in which they would want the questions answered. The questions, which were prepared by a group of middle school teachers, consisted of:

"What is cystic fibrosis?"
"How would a child with cystic fibrosis affect me and my family?"

"What are my chances of being a carrier for cystic fibrosis?"
"Could my developing baby be tested for cystic fibrosis during pregnancy?"
"Is there a way to avoid having a child with cystic fibrosis?"
"What are my chances of having a child with cystic fibrosis?"
"What is cystic fibrosis carrier testing?"

Holtzman and his coworkers found that the order in which patients with and without a family history of CF wanted their questions answered was the same. However, the order in which health care professionals predicted that consumers would want their questions answered was significantly different from that which consumers reported. "We concluded that physicians are not always correct in knowing what their patients want," said Holtzman.

What then, do consumers want? Jayne Mackta, of the Alliance of Genetic Support Groups, spoke at the first meeting about consumer needs and partnerships between consumers and health care professionals. Mackta says that in genetics, a person with a "bad" gene is considered part of the problem. Individuals from families with genetic disease may be reluctant to undergo testing when there is no cure or treatment for their disease out of a reluctance to be stigmatized. Mackta conducted a survey of people from all over the country affected by genetic disease and asked them what they wanted in terms of genetic services.

"They want something to fix it—they want a cure, a treatment," said Mackta. "They want someone to answer the question, Why did it happen to me? Many with children who are dying of debilitating chronic disease wanted advice on day-to-day coping. They want a way to confront their pain, anger, fear, guilt, grief, and frustration. They need help in learning to accept the loss of a dream, the shattering of a myth—that if you're good and do the right thing you're going to grow up and everything is going to come out just fine. They need help accepting the fact that for some questions there are no answers, and for some questions there are too many answers."

Perhaps ironically, consumers, particularly those affected by genetic disease, seem to want many of the services provided by geneticists and genetic counselors. They want help in learning to cope. They want continued support, and information to help them choose a suitable course of action, according to Mackta's survey. But at the same time, as Schneider and others have found, they are reluctant to undergo genetic testing, to be reduced to a circle on the pedigree chart.

The greatest challenge for geneticists, genetic counselors, and other health care professionals may be to convince the public—or at least those at risk for genetic disease—of the benefits not necessarily of testing, but of genetic counseling and other services. Once that is accomplished and the demand for genetic services increases, health care professionals face an even greater challenge: to provide genetic services in such a way that the emphasis is on education, counseling, and continued support. Unfortunately, with a paucity of professionals trained to deliver the continuum of genetic services, patients may find a plethora of genetic tests offered with few support services available.

Incorporation of Genetics into Primary Care Services

The notion that all of the genes in the human genome will someday be identified seemed at one time to be the stuff of science fiction; but all of a sudden, 2005, the year in which Francis Collins, Director of the National Human Genome Research Institute, predicts that all human genes will at least be mapped or identified, seems very close at hand. Much of the discussion at the Banbury meetings focused on preparing for the future and developing mechanisms for meeting the anticipated demand for genetic services. As James Allen says, the future may be closer than we think.

"We are already incorporating genetic knowledge into the practice of medicine," says Allen. "I recently looked through medical journals and I was astounded by how many of the articles have something to do with genetics. I found a large number of articles in journals for family physicians and in dermatology, surgery, ophthalmology, and orthopedic journals, where I never expected to see medical genetics." Allen says that many journal articles discussed the use of genetics as a diagnostic tool. "However, treatment and therapy are not too far down the road."

In addition to journal articles, Allen says that evidence of genetics in mainstream medicine abounds. "We're seeing genetics being incorporated into practice throughout all systems of care—not just in isolated instances," he says. "But we need to lay out the concept of primary care and how genetic services fit in. What is the role of primary care practitioners, nurses, genetic counselors? What information needs to get out to the general public? We will be challenged to look broadly at what primary care is. What is it that the primary care practitioner does with a patient and family?"

Allen says that health care providers need education and guidance in understanding not only the scientific advances in genetics, but also the way medicine is practiced as genetics moves to the forefront of health care. "We have a massive education effort before us," he says. "Rarely has there been so much new knowledge as we are seeing now and can expect in the next decade. It cuts across all disciplines. There are changes in the practice environment. But we aren't certain what messages ought to be delivered."

A major goal of the Banbury meetings is to develop a plan for incorporating genetic services into primary care settings. An important aspect of developing such a plan will be to evaluate what is already being done and to draw on the successes and learn from the failures. During the first meeting, participants heard about a successful attempt to integrate genetic services into a community health care environment at the Chinatown Health Clinic in

New York City. Another successful story comes from a rural outreach program in upstate New York. At the second meeting, Sue Pauker, a geneticist at the Harvard Community Health Plan, discussed her organization's success in developing a genetics program in a managed care setting. Drawing on these examples, participants discussed some of the hurdles involved and key elements needed to move genetics into mainstream medicine.

Service Models: How Genetic Services Are Currently Provided

Genetic services are currently delivered in many different types of settings—from academic centers, commercial laboratories, rural outreach programs, community hospitals, managed health care organizations, public health clinics, and private practice. All models of service provide care for different populations and are needed in today's health care environment. If the future does indeed call for an increased need for genetic services, many of these services will have to be provided by primary care practitioners and other health care professionals. The following current practices and programs might serve as models to the general practitioner.

COMMUNITY OUTREACH CENTERS

The Chinatown Health Clinic, which opened in 1992 largely to accommodate a rising immigrant population from Asia, serves as a model system for integrating genetics with primary care services. The clinic operates in full cooperation with, and with the support of, the Divisions of Human Genetics and of Pediatric Hematology at Cornell University Medical College in New York. Bruce Haas, a genetic counselor at the clinic, and Grace Wang, a primary care practitioner and administrator of the clinic, both participated in the first Banbury conference. The clinic is a community center that serves the local Chinatown population—primarily Asian-Americans. The clinic is a primary health care facility providing prenatal care, pediatrics, family medicine, dentistry, and ophthalmology. The clinic is open 7 days per week. Most patients are new to the United States—85% have been in this country for less than 5 years.

According to Wang, most visitors to the Chinatown clinic are from China, in the heart of the so-called thalassemia belt. Thalassemia is a genetic disorder affecting the red blood cells, found most commonly among Italians, Greeks, Asians, and Africans. The disease, characterized by a severe anemia, is caused by a decreased production of one or more of the globin protein chains that form hemoglobin, the oxygen-transporting substance present in the red blood cells. Two major forms of thalassemia are caused by deficiencies in different protein chains. α-Thalassemia is found most often among people from Southeast Asia. Severe forms of α-thalassemia can result in the death of an infant, whereas milder forms can result in chronic anemia or produce no evident signs of disease in asymptomatic carriers. β-Thalassemia is found in two forms, major and minor. The major form, also known as Cooley's anemia, is detected after birth and is characterized by enlarged bones, liver, and spleen. There is no cure, and the only treatment is frequent blood transfusion. Thalassemia major patients rarely live past the age of 20. Most patients with β-thalassemia minor are asymptomatic, but they may pass the abnormal gene for the disease on to offspring. In both α- and β-thalassemia, the more severe forms of the disease are caused by inheriting two altered forms of globin genes (homozygotes), and the milder forms are due to the inheritance of only one altered globin gene (heterozygotes).

A major thrust of the genetic services provided at the Chinatown Health Clinic is to screen patients as carriers for thalassemia both before and after conception. The goals of the screening program include assessing the incidence of α- and β-thalassemia, providing genetic counseling to carriers, and providing prenatal diagnosis to pregnant couples identified as carriers.

The genetic services program at the Chinatown Health Clinic has been well-received in the community, in large part because of the effort to educate both staff and patients about genetics. This includes an effort to integrate genetics education into the training curriculum for all staff members. "The importance of a team approach cannot be underestimated," says Wang. "Each person on the staff represents the clinic, including both medical practitioners and support staff. The front desk clerk has to understand what's going on to screen and direct incoming calls and inquiries."

Haas and Wang say that even drawing blood presents a challenge. "Patients see blood as a life force," says Wang. "They are hesitant to have their blood drawn. We have to explain why it is important."

Wang says that in addition to training staff members, the clinic also tries to educate the public about topical issues in genetics. "We buy air time on Chinese radio and provide information on genetics and other health issues," says Wang. "We also offer a variety of educational pamphlets and brochures describing some of the services."

Haas says it is important to understand the values and culture of the patients. Because so many patients at the clinic are new to the United States, the clinic provides services and information in the patients' native language, primarily Chinese. "We try to instill that they have choices," says Haas. "They are hesitant to challenge authority. Patients at the clinic also have a different concept of fate, which is an important concept in genetic counseling. We have to appreciate that."

THE HARVARD COMMUNITY HEALTH PLAN

Susan Pauker is the executive director of the Harvard Community Health Plan (HCHP) Foundation and the chief of medical genetics at HCHP, a not-for-profit prepaid group health practice involved in teaching, research, and community service.

"We have developed an active genetic services program in the context of a prepaid health plan," says Pauker. "We're hoping to avoid a situation where a 20-year-old comes in 23 weeks pregnant saying 'My father has polycystic kidney disease. Should I be worried about that?'"

In a managed care environment, says Pauker, patients and providers have ready access to geneticists and are able to receive training and educational materials in a familiar setting. The genetics department provides updates on clinical genetics to primary care providers on a regular basis, and teaches genetics to new obstetricians and other physicians who join the plan. The department also conducts on-line searches and telephone consults for providers and provides public education in genetics through a member newsletter. In addition, the HCHP runs a cancer risk assessment clinic and offers preconceptual counseling to all patients.

"A main advantage to the managed care setting is that we can reach patients during the preconception period," says Pauker. "We are missing that opportunity nationally. We take the attitude of caring for a patient for their life, which provides continuity in care." Pauker says that HCHP maintains files on patients with family histories of genetic disease. "When the gene for cystic fibrosis was discovered, we pulled 40 people out of our files and offered testing on the spot. That's the advantage of the system."

Pauker also says that managed care systems may be able to preempt direct targeting of consumers and practitioners by companies hawking DNA tests. "Companies have been hitting on patients and providers directly," says Pauker. "It's possible a pediatrician would release the results of such a test without a protocol for providing counseling. But we have a standard protocol for handling this."

One of the issues in introducing genetics in a primary care setting concerns costs, says Pauker, a sentiment echoed by many meeting participants. Many HMOs and insurance programs may fail to see a cost-savings benefit associated with genetic services. Pauker said she started her tenure at HCHP as a pediatrician and later developed the genetics program. "It evolved over time until it became part of the fabric of the program. Now it is clear that you need genetics and that it can decrease costs." Pauker says that as genetics is used more in internal medicine as a diagnostic tool, the long-term cost-savings benefits will be better appreciated. "Genetics will be legitimized when we begin to see it as part of mainstream adult medicine," she says. However, she acknowledges that many for-profit managed care organizations have a higher patient turnover and may be more interested in short-term rather than long-term benefits.

RURAL OUTREACH GENETIC SERVICES

Luba Djurdjinovic, a medical geneticist at the Genetic Counseling Program in Binghamton, New York, oversees a rural outreach project in the

Adirondack Mountains of upstate New York. She finds that practitioners in such environments have to deal with many unique problems not encountered in urban settings.

Djurdjinovic says that a key to the success of her outreach program was the recruitment of two nurses who were members of the local community. The nurses spent the first year of the project assessing whether an outreach project was appropriate. "We let the community determine with us if this was something that they wanted," says Djurdjinovic. "Because the outreach workers were members of the community, I think the energy they put toward getting services out were enhanced rather than would be the case in recruiting an outsider, who would first have to learn about the community."

Several specific beliefs are commonly held in rural communities, says Djurdjinovic. For example, individuals affected by genetic disease are not usually immediately concerned about their condition. "These families are survivors," says Djurdjinovic. "Many families will wait for two years on a waiting list rather than travel to get services they need."

In addition, many rural clients equate genetic services with abortion, eugenics, and research and they are concerned that they will serve as some sort of guinea pig. Rural clients, like their urban and suburban counterparts, perceive no need for services unless they are suggested by the primary care provider.

"We can't just go in and pull people into a clinic," say Djurdjinovic. "But if we have the support of the provider and nurse, there is a continuum of care and people are more eager to participate."

Djurdjinovic says that the continuing education of nursing staff and other community health professionals is critical to the success of the program. "Community and professional education can vary," she says. "But it should be specific to what interests the community. Last year we focused on educating dental hygienists, who very often will make recommendations to patients."

It is also important to be sensitive to family beliefs, according to Djurdjinovic. "People make decisions based on their beliefs. We can't go in there and say that what they believe is not true."

Djurdjinovic says that rural workers also face some practical problems that are not always taught in medical school and professional graduate schools. "Weather is a big problem," said Djurdjinovic. "We don't do any active outreach in January and February. We hibernate. The tremendous distances that have to be covered create logistical problems for both patients and practitioners. People tend to be clustered in small communities and there isn't much in between."

Another major problem in rural programs is confidentiality. A post office in the middle of a grocery store may appear rather benign, but personal letters are typically piled up on the countertop for all to peruse. "Mrs. Smith who lives next door would love to look through your mail, as well," says

Djurdjinovic. "So we have to be careful what appears as the return address."

Finally, says Djurdjinovic, it is important to have an ongoing process of evaluation. "We are now using focus groups to determine what changes need to made in the program. They will tell you what they think. It's really humbling."

Djurdjinovic says that as a director of rural services, she is always on the lookout for innovative solutions to problems. She predicts that technological innovations could revolutionize genetic services in rural communities. For example, at an outreach program based in Columbus, Ohio, a telecommunications system was recently installed that enabled genetic counselors to communicate with clients in rural settings. "This system allows clients, practitioners, and geneticists to have joint consultations," she says. "Such a system could serve people who can't get to service centers."

PRIVATE GENETIC SERVICES

As more and more genes that predispose individuals to disease are discovered, more genetic tests are apt to find their way to the commercial market, and laboratory testing in private settings is bound to increase. Joseph Schulman, a physician and researcher with training in medical genetics, is the founder and current director of the Genetics and IVF Institute in Fairfax, Virginia. Schulman says there are several types of commercial ventures involved in genetic testing:

- *Large industrial enterprises* operated and controlled by large corporations focus on processing a high volume of laboratory tests. Such ventures, which depend on profits to sustain growth, often buy out smaller pathology and genetics testing laboratories. With the advent of managed care, Schulman predicts that such enterprises will be strengthened as they "bid to outdo each other at the lowest price."

- *Venture capitalists* presented as biotechnology companies or spin-offs are unable to compete with large pathology companies.

- *Integrated high-care laboratories*, which are owned by the providers of service, feature extensive contacts between providers and patients receiving genetic services.

- *Small, genetic service organizations* in the community rarely generate sufficient capital to be self-sustaining.

- *University hospitals and affiliated laboratories* are often indistinct from private laboratories. Sometimes professionals associated with such laboratories can direct specimens for testing at self-owned private laboratories.

Presently, most genetic testing carried out in commercial laboratories is cytogenetic analysis—the testing of chromosome and cellular abnormalities—and does not include an analysis of the DNA sequence or mutations in the sequence. Schulman says that as the DNA-based tests become more routine, it will be difficult to predict which types of commercial laboratories will have the most success. He predicts that as the health care system moves toward managed care, many private laboratories, including the Genetics and IVF Institute, will try to integrate services into a primary care model.

Many are concerned that the commercial market will drive the perceived "need" for genetic testing and that the government should more closely regulate the services offered by private laboratories. However, Schulman says that tight regulation may not be necessary. "You can't build a program or company on something that's not real," he says. "You can't fool large numbers of people, if you don't have a good product to begin with." Others contend that in the area of genetics in which provider and the public have absorbed little information, they can easily be fooled. Consequently, regulation of genetic services is needed.

COMMUNITY HOSPITAL-BASED GENETIC SERVICES

Nancy Fisher is a medical geneticist who works through two community-based hospitals in Seattle, Washington, in both urban and rural environments. Fisher finds that her biggest hurdle in both the urban and rural settings is the reluctance of hospital personnel to resort to utilizing genetic services. "Many urban hospitals would rather use a cookbook approach to diagnosing genetic conditions," says Fisher. "They prefer ordering an ultrasound examination to conducting a genetic test. They will rely on genetics only as a last resort."

Fisher says that typically, a physician will refer a patient to a medical geneticist for diagnostic purposes, but usually the patients will first see a genetic counselor. "We operate on a triage system," says Fisher. "After consulting with a genetic counselor a patient may be referred to me to help with the diagnosis."

In the urban community hospital setting, Fisher primarily sees patients seeking prenatal and neonatal diagnoses, including patients with hemoglobinopathies, as well as a growing number of adult cancer patients. In the rural setting, where her patients are primarily children, she is frequently consulted to diagnose patients with fetal alcohol syndrome. Fisher says that hospitals in both the urban and rural environments are reluctant to embrace genetics. "Hospitals see genetic counseling as a labor-intensive service that doesn't pull in money," Fisher said at the meeting. "It will be even more difficult for genetics to find a niche in the managed health care setting." Fisher says that a major challenge for geneticists is to convince them that in the long run, genetic testing is a cost-effective system for screening patients and preventing disease.

GENETIC SERVICES TARGETED TO SINGLE-GENE DISORDERS

Medical professionals without intensive training in human genetics may feel unprepared to take on the role of genetic counselors for the seemingly infinite spectrum of genetic diseases. However, for genetic diseases that are caused by mutations in a single gene and have a high incidence in specific racial or ethnic groups, training in genetics may be relatively straightforward. Non-geneticists may be able to play a vital role in delivering genetic services for single-gene disorders such as sickle cell anemia, thalassemia, and cystic fibrosis, according to Doris Wethers, a medical geneticist at St. Luke's Roosevelt Hospital Center in New York City. The screening for the related genetic disorders—known collectively as hemoglobinopathies—that are caused by mutations in the globin genes and affect the production of hemoglobin in the red blood cells, may serve as a good model system for screening for other types of single-gene disorders.

In the early 1970s, researchers developed rapid, inexpensive tests for diagnosing sickle cell anemia and other hemoglobinopathies, which were rapidly implemented in the African-American community. Many community-based organizations with large numbers of clients quickly evolved. Eventually, many of these single-gene screening programs were integrated into state-run genetic services. "Many of these programs withered and died on the vine," said Wethers at the Banbury meeting. "There were no more sickle cell clinics to give total counseling to the community at large."

Through more recent newborn screening programs, thousands of families have been identified as carriers of sickle cell anemia, says Wethers. However, these screening programs do not include a mandate to conduct genetic counseling, and the issue of whether other family members should be notified remains controversial.

"What are we going to do with the large number of carriers who have been identified through screening programs?" she asks. "There aren't enough counselors available to reach and adequately counsel these families."

Wethers says that the need for genetic counselors is particularly acute in many southern states, where the population of African-Americans is large. For example, although 177 genetic counselors practice in California, currently only 2 master's-level genetic counselors are certified to practice in Mississippi.

Wethers says that the genetic counseling program at St. Luke's utilizes many non-geneticists to counsel patients for sickle cell anemia. Single-gene counselors are individuals from varied educational backgrounds with specific training in the genetics of one particular condition. Usually single-gene counselors understand the basic patterns of Mendelian inheritance. They are familiar with the symptoms of the disease, and they understand basic genetic principles. In addition, single-gene counselors are well-acquainted with the basic counseling process, according to Wethers. Currently, California and

Massachusetts are the only states that certify counselors for single-gene disorders.

"Much of what we do involves the education of the community at large, as well as counseling and educating the families who come to us at the clinic," she says. "This means going out into community, giving presentations, and letting them know what is meant by sickle cell anemia." According to Wethers, all medical personnel—nurses, nurse practitioners, medical social workers, and physicians—conduct both educational and counseling service on a regular basis.

Beyond sickle cell, single-gene counselors could be utilized to counsel for other genetic disorders, thus relieving the burden on master's-level genetic counselors and other health care providers, says Wethers.

Among the advantages of focusing on single-gene counselors is their potential for providing culturally appropriate, sensitive, linguistically compatible counseling, says Wethers. "Currently there is little role for the non-geneticist as a single-gene counselor, but it certainly is an avenue that should be investigated."

CANCER GENETICS

Katherine Schneider, as a genetic counselor at the Dana Farber Cancer Institute in Boston, Massachusetts, conducts cancer risk counseling. Presently, Schneider and her colleagues are evaluating two different models, which test for two different genetic defects, as paradigms for genetic risk counseling. In one system, Schneider and her colleagues counsel patients from families at high risk for Li-Fraumeni syndrome for mutations in the p53 gene. In a second model, the researchers counsel and test patients from families at high risk for breast cancer for mutations in the BRCA1 gene.

Li-Fraumeni is a rare cancer syndrome that occurs in fewer than 300 families in the world. Members of these families are at high risk for developing a host of different cancers, including osteosarcoma, breast cancer, leukemia, and brain tumors. The syndrome appears to be caused by a germ-line mutation in the p53 gene, which codes for a protein that is thought to play a role in DNA repair. As illustrated in a sample pedigree (Fig. 1), a variety of tumors can occur in the same family, and individuals often develop cancer by the age of 30. The lifetime risk for developing cancer is 90%.

To be eligible for the study, patients had to be adult members of a family with a germ-line mutation in the p53 gene, English speaking, and cognitively and emotionally competent. Adhering to counseling procedures developed for the genetic counseling of Huntington's disease, participants were advised to identify a local psychologist, bring a support person to counseling sessions, and agree to a physical examination prior to counseling.

The counseling sessions were conducted in three visits. During the first visit (Pretest), patients met with an oncologist, who discussed the medical im-

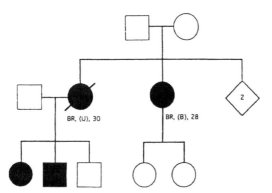

Figure 1 Example of a pedigree with Li-Fraumeni syndrome. Diagnosis (laterality), age at diagnosis; BR, breast cancer; CN, brain tumor; SS, soft tissue sarcoma; OC, osteosarcoma; U, unilateral; B, bilateral; boxed 2, two unaffected siblings, either sex. (Reprinted, with permission, from Schneider 1994.)

plications of testing for the p53 mutation, as well as options available for early detection and prevention of cancer. A genetic counselor was also present to discuss the advantages and disadvantages of testing, as well as implications for the family. For example, some people feel they are better able to cope if they know with greater certainty their risk for developing cancer. Others may be unprepared to cope with the news that they are likely to develop cancer.

During the first visit, patients were invited to submit to a test for p53 mutations. If patients elected to have the test, they would meet with a genetic counselor, oncologist, and psychologist during the second visit. During this session, the oncologist and genetic counselor would discuss test results as well as the implications of these results. The psychologist would assess the immediate reaction of the patients and discuss coping strategies. At a follow-up visit 3 months after the disclosure of test results, patients met with a genetic counselor to discuss early detection and prevention options, and surveillance strategies, and to review information, and with a psychologist to discuss long-term adjustment and coping strategies. As discussed on page 21, none of the patients contacted wanted to be tested, primarily because they were trying to cope with losses in the family.

In a second study, Schneider and her colleagues assessed a model for counseling and testing patients from families at high risk for breast cancer due to mutations in the newly discovered BRCA1 gene. Mutations in the BRCA1 gene are estimated to account for more than half of all inherited breast cancers. The role of BRCA1 in nonheritable forms of breast cancer, which accounts for 90–95% of all breast cancers, remains unclear (see Fig. 2).

As shown above, in families at high risk for breast cancer due to mutations in the BRCA1 gene, individuals tend to develop breast cancer in their 30s and 40s. In some families, there is also a significant risk of ovarian cancer in females and of prostate cancer in males.

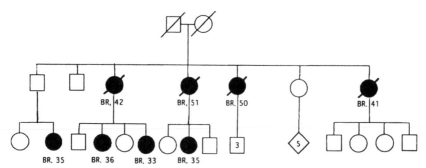

Figure 2 Pedigree of family with early-onset breast cancer. Diagnosis, age at diagnosis; boxed 3, three unaffected brothers; boxed 5, five unaffected siblings of either sex. (Pedigree provided by Dr. Judy E. Garber, Dana-Farber Cancer Institute; reprinted, with permission, from Schneider 1994.)

Schneider and her colleagues offered the test for BRCA1 alterations to affected men and women, unaffected women, women with cancer, and men. For BRCA1 screening, Schneider and her colleagues have opted for a two-visit model. During the first visit, patients meet with a genetic counselor and oncologist, who provide information about breast cancer and the concept of risk, the implications of testing, and the pros and cons of testing. During the second visit, for those who decide to be tested, patients meet with an oncologist, genetic counselor, and a psychologist. During this meeting, the oncologist discloses the test results and discusses the implications. Both the genetic counselor and the oncologist also discuss surveillance options and prevention strategies. The psychologist is also on hand to assess reaction and to discuss coping strategies. So far, Schneider says, 69 individuals have agreed to testing for BRCA1, out of a total of 104 individuals approached.

A major goal of Schneider's program is to evaluate the benefits of genetic screening and counseling for cancer; but not all members of high-risk families are comfortable with the notion of genetic testing. The challenge in such families is to provide all the necessary information to allow individuals to make informed decisions without directly influencing their decision whether or not to be tested.

STATE HEALTH DEPARTMENT-INITIATED GENETIC SERVICES

As both Fisher and Schneider attest, in order for genetic services to catch on, both medical providers and patients must feel comfortable with the concept of genetic services and, when appropriate, genetic testing. One approach to accomplishing this goal is through public education, which, as the Chinatown Health Clinic suggests, plays an important role in gaining patient acceptance.

An approach to educating the public about genetics can occur through public health programs. George Cunningham, of the Genetic Disease branch of the California State Department of Health Services in Berkeley, California, oversees a comprehensive centrally controlled program for public education in California. Cunningham's department offers books, brochures, newsletters, reference manuals, fact sheets, and access to on-line computer databases for both the general public and health professionals. In addition, the department distributes curricula for grades K–12 on genetics. The information provided covers a wide variety of topics, largely focused on prenatal screening for hemoglobinopathies, galactosemia, phenylketonuria (PKU), analysis of alpha-fetoprotein (AFP), and Down's syndrome.

"The most effective education occurs when the provider's patient has a problem," said Cunningham at the Banbury meeting. "That's when individuals [providers and consumers] want information, and they want easy access to the information." Cunningham says that all materials are distributed to the public through the physicians, who are responsible for fully informing their patients of the risks and benefits of any screening or diagnostic procedure. Cunningham and his colleagues have recently developed a computer-based resource center known as GeneHELP, which consists of a database of over 460 titles of material on genetic diseases, hemoglobinopathies, birth defects, newborn screening, and prenatal diagnosis issues. The service will soon be available through the Internet.

GENETIC SERVICES IN AN ACADEMIC HEALTH CENTER

Most genetic counselors and medical geneticists are affiliated with academic health centers. However, within the university setting, a wide spectrum of services are found.

"I don't really think there is an academic model," said Mark Lubinsky, a physician and medical geneticist at the Children's Hospital of Wisconsin in Milwaukee, speaking at the first Banbury meeting. "What is done at any one center depends on the personnel and who is running it. Some centers have a heavy focus on research and provide little service. Some are just the opposite." At Children's Hospital, Lubinsky and his team of geneticists and genetic counselors, in addition to running a general genetics clinic, provide genetic services to patients with sickle cell anemia, hemophilia, and hemoglobinopathies; conduct CF screening programs; and consult with patients and their families who are affected by muscular dystrophy, cleft palate, and neurofibromatosis.

According to Lubinsky, genetic services at university-associated hospitals are prone to some of the same problems that confront private and community-based hospitals, as described by Nancy Fisher. "We should be able to provide all these services, in addition to conducting research, and teaching," says Lubinsky. "And we should be able to do this all profitably."

Unfortunately, says Lubinsky, too much emphasis is placed on profits. "The accomplishments of which I am most proud are not cost-effective," says Lubinsky. "I go in and tell parents that their child will die or that their child will be retarded." In a managed care setting, time devoted to helping patients cope with their diagnoses is not always rewarded, in Lubinsky's opinion. "In a heavily HMOed health care climate, it's cheaper to let people suffer," he says.

Cultural Issues and Ethical Considerations

Geneticists and genetic counselors expressed concern that as genetic services are dispensed by other health care professionals, the goals of the counseling process are maintained. These include ensuring patient confidentiality, delivering information in a culturally sensitive manner, preserving patient autonomy by delivering information in a nondirective way, and obtaining fully informed consent.

Cultural Issues

To understand the importance of culture in providing genetic services, consider the following case scenarios provided by Diana Punales-Morejon, a genetic counselor at Beth Israel Medical Center in New York City.

Case 1: Mr. and Mrs. B. are recent Chinese immigrants to the United States. They have two daughters alive and well and one son who died from a childhood infection in China. Mrs. B. is 34 years old. She was referred for genetic counseling by her obstetrician because of her age-related risk of having a child with a chromosome abnormality. The couple comes for genetic counseling along with the husband's mother. They express an interest in amniocentesis because they have heard that you can learn the sex of the fetus through this test. The mother-in-law is particularly concerned that the couple have a son. Mrs. B clearly expresses that she doesn't think she would keep the pregnancy if it is not a boy.

What counseling approach do we use with this couple? What role do we think the mother-in-law plays in this family? What is the significance of having a male child for this couple? How do we deal with this issue of sex selection?

Case 2: Mr. and Mrs. R. are Latinos from the Dominican Republic. They have been in the United States for 10 years. Because their family is not here, they make frequent trips back and forth. Mrs. R. is a homemaker who raises the couple's four children, two girls and two boys who are alive and well. Mr. R. is self-employed. Mrs. R. is 29 years old and Mr. R. is 35. She was referred to a genetic counselor by her obstetrician because of an abnormal

AFP test result. The couple comes to the office quite upset. They are told that the baby has some problem because of a low protein in the blood. Mrs. R. relates that she is feeling bad because she hasn't been eating well during the pregnancy. Mr. R. completely dominates the session and his wife appears submissive. When the couple is offered amniocentesis, Mr. R. is the one who responds. He states that he doesn't want his wife to have the needle test because it will hurt the baby.

Again, what approach do we use with this couple? How do we think Mrs. R. feels? How do we work with this couple to help them reach a decision about amniocentesis?

Case 3: Mr. and Mrs. S. were referred for genetic counseling by their HMO because Mrs. S. is 37 years old and faces an age-related risk of having a child with a chromosome abnormality. Mrs. S. is African-American and her family is originally from South Carolina. Mr. S.'s family is from the West Indies. He is an attorney and she is a psychologist. During the pregnancy history-taking, Mrs. S. reported that she drinks two glasses of dark beer a day because Mr. S.'s grandmother recommended that this is the best thing for a baby in the West Indies. She followed her advice for her first pregnancy and plans to continue doing so with this one.

What approach do we use with this couple? What significance does beer drinking have for them? How do we tell them about the use of alcohol during pregnancy?

"Cases like these are encountered every day by individuals providing genetic services," says Punales-Morejon. "The genetic needs of the individuals that we serve are determined by our clients' distinct cultural, ethnic, and social background." Punales-Morejon says that at present birth and immigration rates, by the next century, 50% of the U.S. population will be non-white and that by 2056, whites will be a minority.

Genetic counselors deal with diversity and ethnocultural issues every day, says Punales-Morejon. Despite the large numbers of minorities in this country, many geneticists and health care professionals are inadequately prepared to counsel such individuals in the context of their ethnic and cultural backgrounds. "We need to consider how the race, ethnicity, culture and gender affect service delivery," says Punales-Morejon. "The Western model of medicine involves self determination, verbalization, and the revealing of intimacies to strangers. This mode may not be appropriate for all cultures." Failure to appreciate ethnic differences can result in a decreased utilization of services and low-quality care, she says.

Punales-Morejon recommends that genetic counselors, geneticists, and other health professionals strive to:

• utilize a multicultural and multilingual staff

- undergo cultural sensitivity training for staff members

- develop an awareness of biases

- understand the epidemiology of diseases among a particular ethnic group

- realize that disparate care is a reality

Patient Issues

Peppered throughout almost all discussions at the Banbury Center meetings were concerns of preserving patient autonomy—the patient's right to make his or her own decisions. Traditionally, geneticists and genetic counselors attempt to deliver genetic services using a nondirected approach—they provide the client with all the information necessary to make a fully informed consent, but do not themselves recommend or decide on a course of action. Implicit in the process is the notion that patients are made aware of all the pros and cons associated with genetic testing and genetic counseling and that they provide their informed consent prior to utilizing services.

As genetic services move out of the exclusive domain of geneticists and genetic counselors, away from decisions related solely to reproduction and toward assessing an individual's predisposition to adult-onset disease, many wonder whether informed consent will remain the standard or whether health care workers will rely on implied consent—the assumption that the client is consenting to services merely by keeping an appointment.

"As the number of genetic tests increases, as well as the number of individuals providing genetic services, will that necessitate moving from an informed consent to an implied consent model?" asks Phil Reilly. "Is that acceptable?" Reilly says that as genetic services are expanded and more practitioners are trained in genetics, the issue of informed consent will have to be resolved and inculcated into the training curricula.

Another issue for practitioners is that of providing nondirective counseling. Holtzman is particularly concerned that physicians will have an especially difficult time refraining from telling their patients what decisions to make. He has conducted a survey of primary care practitioners to assess their attitudes toward directed versus nondirected counseling.

In that study, Holtzman and his colleagues surveyed medical practitioners from different disciplines and, based on protocols for testing for CF carrier status, asked survey respondents whether they would tell a high-risk couple what to do about prenatal diagnosis. "Among genetic counselors, 100% would not give their own opinion when counseling the couple," said Holtzman. "Among medical geneticists, 85% would withhold their own opinion. But only about 50% of practitioners in other specialties would not give an opinion. And some will tell a patient outright what to do." In addition, Holtzman's group found that female physicians were less likely than males to offer their own opinion.

"Physicians say that their patients want to hear their opinions," says Holtzman, but he contends that many physicians do not know what their patients want. In another study, Holtzman and his colleagues found that physicians did not accurately predict the information to which their clients wanted access.

"Patients are not taking an active enough role in making decisions about their own care," says Holtzman. "I have had to suggest to my own relatives who are not in the medical field, what questions to ask their doctors. Part of the thrust in efforts to educate the public and professionals about genetics might include information on preserving or instilling patient autonomy," he says.

If genetic services are ever to be fully embraced by the public at large, or within families at risk for genetic disease, then the privacy of genetic information is vital. Individuals may be reluctant to submit to genetic tests and other genetic services if the information will become part of their health record, to which insurance companies and employers may have access. Meeting participants discussed the need for assurances for the privacy of genetic information, although exactly how this will be guaranteed remains a point of contention. Insurance companies hold that as long as a patient has access to any health information, so too should they. Ultimately, this problem will be addressed through legislation at both the state and national level. Indeed, several bills addressing different aspects of privacy of genetic information have been introduced in Congress.

Who Will Provide Genetic Services?

The numbers speak for themselves. Millions and millions of people throughout this country alone are affected by genetic disease, either as carriers, family members, or patients. Yet, there are fewer than 2000 professionals specifically trained to provide genetic services. Clearly, help is needed.

Professionals from several health disciplines are well-positioned to provide at least some basic genetic services, if properly trained. Family physicians, pediatricians, obstetricians, internists, nurses, nurse practitioners, physicians' assistants, and social workers constitute a large reservoir of untapped talent that could help relieve a large part of the genetic crunch. Even lay personnel, such as health educators, could serve as counselors for single-gene disorders.

Social Workers

Medical social workers at the master's degree level complete course work in human behavior, policy, research, individual, family, and group practice counseling and therapy, advocacy and case management. Medical social workers practice in primary health care settings, in mental health, in child welfare settings, and substance abuse programs, as well as in public agencies and in private practice. However, the integration of genetics into social work has not been overwhelmingly successful. Part of the problem in training social workers in genetics is a matter of habit, and part is due to a difference in outlook between the two disciplines, according to Rita Beck-Black, a social worker with training in genetic counseling, of Columbia University in New York. "It's hard for social workers to own genetics as central to what we are about," said Beck at the Banbury meeting. "Diversity and culture have been mandated into the curriculum." It's difficult to reconcile that philosophy with a genetic perspective, she says.

Practical issues also prevent genetics from gaining ground among social workers. Few faculty have the background and knowledge in genetics to integrate it into the existing curricula. In addition, master's programs in social work already cover a wide range and great volume of material, and universities are hesitant to add more. "Change comes slowly to academia," says Beck-Black.

Beck-Black says that increasing access to genetic information is crucial to training social workers in genetics. She suggests developing training models for social workers that are specifically linked to the concerns of social workers. A short-term goal, she says, is providing opportunities in continuing education for genetics training. "Continuing education is an immediate priority," says Beck-Black. "This provides the most flexible and open-ended opportunity for making changes." Although schools of social work are slow to change, she nevertheless supports efforts to develop new genetics curricula for schools of social work and suggests linking genetics education to existing courses.

Beck-Black points out that social workers have experience in one aspect of counseling that may be useful in a population mistrustful of genetics research. "We are often faced with the question, How do we offer service to someone who doesn't want it?" she says. "Our primary responsibility is to help the client. We have a responsibility to minimize harm, and we often have to juggle protections."

Nurses

Many surveys have shown that nurses are interested in genetic services, says Anne Matthews, a nurse by training who runs the master's program in genetic counseling at the University of Colorado in Denver. According to Matthews, nurses already provide many components of genetic services. These include identifying families at risk, reviewing family histories, identifying risk factors, providing referrals for families needing genetic services, telling patients and families what they might expect, and reinforcing genetic information after referral. Nurses, because they are in frequent contact with patients, can be important in the follow-up phases of genetic services. They help families cope and serve as patient advocates. These are all services that tend to fall by the wayside. However, most nurses do not have the genetic framework and knowledge in genetics to enhance the provision of genetic services.

Matthews predicts that as health care funds decrease, those in primary care roles will take over some of the specialists' roles, particularly in single-gene counseling. "It's important that nurses and other primary care providers have the education base to know when to refer out—when a particular case doesn't fit the mold."

Physicians

According to James Allen of the American Medical Association, primary care physicians will play a vital role in the delivery of genetic services. Obstetricians, pediatricians, and family medicine practitioners in particular may serve as valuable resources in providing patients with genetic information. "Primary care physicians serve an important function as coordinators of health care delivery," said Allen at the Banbury meeting. "Primary care physicians are concerned with the whole person."

Allen predicts that the role of the physician in the delivery of traditional genetic services, such as screening for classic, inherited diseases, is unlikely to change significantly. "But in other areas, there will be enormous changes as the Human Genome Project provides more information on genes," he says. "Many medical conditions with simple or complex relationships to gene alleles will arise. There will be a lot of hype, and test availability may present an enormous problem." For example, the relationship between a genetic mutation, disease, penetrance, prevalence in different population groups, and steps to prevention are all areas that physicians must be able to discuss with their patients.

Training physicians in genetics will present some unique challenges, says Allen. "Many physicians will embrace the new developments, some may avoid them," he says. "There is a great need for accurate information. But beyond that, physicians will have a hard time being nondirective, relying on counselors, or using a team approach."

Preserving a Niche for Genetic Service Professionals

An underlying theme throughout the course of the Banbury Center meeting was concern over the future role of geneticists and genetic counselors in a managed care setting. Clearly, genetic counselors have more business than they can currently handle. Therefore, genetic counselors and geneticists are being asked to help impart genetic information to the primary care practitioners. However, according to some meeting attendees, HMOs and managed care facilities have little use for genetic counselors. Many genetics professionals fear they will be pushed out of the very field they have worked hard at establishing.

What then will become of geneticists and genetic counselors? Will their numbers increase until they are a commonplace fixture in HMOs? Will they remain in academic settings, setting the standards for genetic counseling practice? Or will they become obsolete as genetic counseling services are increasingly provided by other health practitioners?

Most health care professionals believe that there will be a place for everyone, as genetic information continues to expand exponentially. "In talks with managed care organizations I'm told that there will be a paradigm shift," says Mark Lubinsky, a medical geneticist. "This may present a challenge or an opportunity for geneticists and genetic counselors as we find our way in the system. But we need to be proactive."

Goals: Delivery of Genetic Services

Geneticists, genetic counselors, primary care physicians, and nurses may indeed have different ideas about how to best incorporate genetics into primary care practice. Genetic counselors, for example, are more inclined to emphasize some of the human and ethical issues as top priorities. They cite community involvement, communication skills, cultural sensitivity, gaining patient trust, and maintaining patient privacy and autonomy as important considerations. Primary care physicians may have more concerns about some of the more practical issues: how to get access to needed information, how to arrange for payment for services, and how to develop standards of care, for example.

There is also some common ground. All groups of health care providers seem to agree that the effort will require a multipronged approach that incorporates all of these facets. Mechanisms for ensuring adequate and ongoing education of health care professionals, developing a team approach to service delivery, developing methods for evaluating service delivery, providing safeguards for protecting against discrimination, and maintaining cultural sensitivity are all goals cited at both meetings that need to be kept up front. Although geneticists, genetic counselors, physicians, and nurses may place different emphases on some priorities, there appears to be general agreement on what aspects need to be considered as genetics moves into mainstream health care. Among the essential steps to ease the shift of genetics into primary care, Banbury conference participants cited several key considerations :

- *Primary care providers.* Recognize that primary care providers include physicians in family medicine, internal medicine, pediatrics, and OB/GYN, as well as community health nurses, nurse midwives, nurse practitioners, public health nurses, and physician's assistants. Define the expectations, roles, and responsibilities of each. What do primary care providers expect of genetic specialists and vice versa? Collect data to determine whether there is a deficiency or maldistribution of genetic services, and identify areas of need.

- *Family doctor/primary practitioner.* Establish communication with primary practitioners who serve the local community, making every effort to provide educational material and training in genetics education.

- *Consumers of genetic services.* Identify the consumers of genetic services. Will they be defined as those affected by a genetic disorder or as the public at large? Assess what services are needed in the population and what expectations exist among consumers, patients, and payers. Involve consumer groups in dispensing information about new services and tests as they become available.

- *Community involvement.* Involve members of the local community in all stages of genetic service delivery. This can include local input into determining what the community wants and needs, planning the implementation of services, and training local community members to deliver services.

- *Standards of care.* Develop standards and a process of care for clinical genetics. This should include the identification of clinical indicators, standards for genetic testing, development of a family history tool, the development of algorithms for specific genetic diseases, and the evaluation of the appropriateness of nondirective counseling.

- *Evaluation.* Provide for ongoing, continual evaluation, involving the community whenever possible. This should include both long-term and short-term effects of genetic services, including psychological and quality-of-life considerations. Establish databases, networks, resources, and alliances to improve quality and availability of services, based on outcomes.

- *Cost/benefit analysis.* Assess the needs of consumers and practitioners. Collect data to determine the cost benefit and cost effectiveness of services. The question of how resources for genetic services should be allocated must be addressed. Does the delivery of genetic service leave society better off compared with alternative uses of resources?

- *Cultural sensitivity.* Be aware of the customs, values, and literacy levels as well as the ethnic and cultural differences of the local community and families. Recognize the context in which genetic services are received. Provide services in native languages.

- *Staff training.* Train all staff members, including support staff members, to be comfortable with a basic understanding of genetics and genetic disease. Provide continuing education to increase base level of knowledge, keeping current with new discoveries.

- *Team approach.* Recognize the unique contributions of all members of the health care team and capitalize on complementary talents of personnel. Primary care providers should be the first contact for patients seeking genetic services and education. Genetics in primary care practice should rely on opportunities providing continuity of care and integration of services.

- *Single-gene counselors.* Consider developing a cadre of counselors for genetic conditions caused by a single gene. If appropriate, train non-geneticist personnel to counsel for single-gene disorders. This may relieve the burden placed on geneticists and genetic counselors.

- *Attention to details.* Recognize that small inconveniences can make big differences in the delivery of genetic services, from concerns over having nosy neighbors reading the return address on mail, to inaccessible roadways.

Hurdles

Although many types of genetic services are now commonplace, several issues need to be addressed before genetic services and genetic testing based on advances in genetics research make their way into mainstream health care. Some issues that arose throughout discussions of service models include:

- *Access to care.* Preexisting clauses to specific illnesses prevent coverage and access to care under many health plans. Many individuals still lack coverage for basic health care services. Before patients can have access to genetic services, access to basic health care must first be ensured. Access to care must also be ensured as people move and change jobs or life situations. A portable health record is also needed to ensure that appropriate services are delivered.

- *Gaining patient trust.* Many patients and families are inherently mistrustful of new ideas and technologies. Innovative strategies for building trust between geneticists and local communities need to be devised.

- *Understanding of the Human Genome Project.* In addition to establishing trust on a personal level, many individuals mistrust and misunderstand the purpose of the Human Genome Project. Strategies for public education about the HGP as well as the basics of human genetics and genetic disease, require further consideration.

- *Integrating genetic counseling and managed health care.* Genetic services are perceived as unprofitable. Long-term benefits of genetic services, such as avoiding unnecessary medical procedures, need to be conveyed. Innovative strategies for finding a niche for genetics in managed health care deserve special attention.

- *Privacy issues.* Mechanisms for ensuring that genetic information remains confidential have been widely discussed, but the issue remains unresolved. Legislation may be needed to prevent discrimination and protect privacy, especially in health insurance.

- *Reimbursement issues.* For services to continue and survive, the services must be billed to and reimbursed by third-party payers. Reimbursement must be correlated with the services provided. This should include procedures, cognitive services, and counseling.

- *Different points of view.* According to William Freeman, as genetics moves into mainstream medicine, it is clear that geneticists and primary care practitioners sometimes speak a different language, or at least have a different approach to treating patients:

	Genetic providers	*Primary care providers*
How to do the work	Tend to do history, diagnosis and treatment all in 1 visit	Tend to stretch treatment (and sometimes history and diagnosis) over several visits
What work is done	Prefer to deal with only genetics	Tend to combine gender/age counseling with other gender/age-specific tasks
Length of the visit	1–2 hours	12–30 minutes
Definitiveness of diagnosis and treatment	Want definitive diagnosis and treatment within the visit	More tentative; often let "tincture of time" help the diagnosis and treatment declare itself
Counseling	Pretest counseling as important as or more important than posttest counseling	Posttest more important than than pretest counseling; assume that the patient needs to get the information of the test to be informed enough to make a posttest decision
Nondirective	In every genetics situation, as unlimited and absolute value	Value is partial and limited in most situations (more true in family medicine, general internal medicine, obstetrics and gynecology; less in pediatrics; least in nurse practitioner, certified nurse midwife)

Predictive value of screening patients by the provider	Higher, because many patients and families have been "pre-screened" so that many have genetic disease	Lower, because there is no "pre-screening" to increase predictive value; try to look for ways that are inexpensive in time and money to pre-screen
Severity of genetic disease	More severe, due to preselection of more severe patients and not doing diagnostic workups in the general population	Less severe, due to referral or self-referral of more severe patients, and seeing those patients in the general population with fewer symptoms
Referrals	Some in the genetics community believe in seeing every patient and assuming charge of the more complex cases	Some in the primary care community believe in referring only those we feel we feel cannot handle and co-managing some of even the most complex cases
Anticipatory guidance preventive counseling	Emphasized, but in families with disease, around the time they are identified	Emphasized, but in the context of general life counseling (i.e., during the appropriate stratified preventive services or anticipatory guidance)

How Will Genetic Service Providers Be Trained?

Organizers of the Banbury Center meetings stated: There is a growing body of genetic information—more than service providers can handle. What impact does that have on primary health care providers? What do providers need to know and how can that information be conveyed to them?

Because geneticists and genetic counselors cannot fulfill all the needs for genetic services, they must meet the challenge of educating other health care professionals to counsel patients at risk for genetic disorders. "If I couldn't do what I do now, how could I turn this over to a primary health care specialist?" asked genetic counselor Ann Walker. "What mechanism might we come up with to transfer this knowledge? What might primary care providers want to do?" It is unlikely that any one system will be effective for training all the personnel needed to deliver genetic information to patients and their families, but several programs in effect throughout the country may serve as models for educating nurses, primary care practitioners, and other health professionals.

The first Banbury meeting focused primarily on information that geneticists and genetic counselors would like to convey to practitioners to help them deliver genetic services. Models for continuing education, professional outreach, and specific educational initiatives were discussed. During the second meeting, attended largely by primary care practitioners and policymakers, discussion focused on the information that primary practitioners would like to know in order to provide genetic services and how to get this information infused into medical and nursing school curricula.

Attitudes among Health Care Professionals

As a starting point in integrating genetics into the health care system, it is essential to understand the attitudes toward genetics that exist among health care professionals, who will be the main conveyors of genetics information to the general public and health care consumer. With this in mind, Neil Holtzman conducted a survey of invitees to the second meeting, most of whom are involved in health care in some capacity. The purpose of the study was to assess the needs and interests of those who play a role in health care delivery and education. Such information will be helpful not only in developing appropriate educational materials and curricula for primary care practitioners, but also for developing model systems of care in delivering genetic information in the primary health care setting, according to Holtzman. Details of this survey can be found on pages 79–86.

In addition, the American Nurses Association has conducted a study of attitudes toward genetics, and Holtzman has also conducted a study of physicians' attitudes toward genetics and genetic services. The results of these studies are summarized below.

NURSES: ATTITUDES AND KNOWLEDGE

As a first step toward preparing nurses to provide genetic services in some capacity, the American Nurses Association, based in Washington, D.C., conducted a recent survey to assess the knowledge base and attitudes toward genetics among members of the nursing profession. At the Banbury Center meeting, Colleen Scanlon, director of the ANA's center on Ethics and Human Rights, discussed the goals of the grant project that was funded by the NIH Human Genome Project. According to Scanlon, the project on "Managing Genetic Information: Implications for Nursing Practice" has three main goals:

- to understand the experience of nurses related to eliciting, transferring, and using genetic information in their work with clients and their families

- to identify ethical dilemmas and situations that nurses face during the course of their work

- to develop resources to assist nurses in managing the challenges that accompany advances in genetics

Scanlon surveyed 1000 nurses selected randomly from the membership of the ANA about their attitudes, concerns, and experiences with genetics in their practice. Initially, Scanlon included questions in the survey designed to assess the state of content knowledge in genetics among practicing nurses. However, when piloted, the survey questions related to content were difficult for respondents to answer and affected their desire to engage in the completion of the survey.

Scanlon then revised the survey and excluded questions related to genetic knowledge. "We realized that it was probably true that nurses didn't have that grounding in genetics and that there was no need to build a piece of that into the survey," says Scanlon. "We wanted to be sure to get the information that we really wanted, which was, Is this impacting your practice at all? If it is, are you feeling prepared to deal with it? If not, how can we better prepare you?" Scanlon obtained an 88% response rate with the revised survey.

Of the nurses surveyed, 25% reported a family history of a genetic disorder or condition. Seventy-two percent had children, of which 11% have a genetic disorder. Approximately 25% of the nurses reported that they have a family history of genetic conditions or disorders. All of the survey respondents were involved in direct client care. The majority of the respondents (71%) reported working a mean of 28 hours per week. Most (73%) worked in a hospital setting and over half (64%) identified themselves as a staff nurse while 9% held head nurse, assistant head nurse, or nurse supervisor positions, 7% were clinical specialists, and 5% were nurse practitioners. Of the sample, 25% reported providing direct client care in both ambulatory care and inpatient settings. The ambulatory care settings included hospital outpatient settings, clinics or health departments, group and solo practices, and HMOs. The remainder of the nurses worked in other settings such as mental health, school health, and home health care. Respondents reported providing care for clients with medical/surgical, pediatric, obstetrical/gynecological, orthopedic, neurologic, and cardiac conditions.

Scanlon found that although the respondents worked in varied clinical settings with different educational backgrounds, and that many had firsthand experience with genetic disease, only 9% had ever had a formal course in genetics! In fact, only 15% reported that a genetics course was even offered during their education. Survey respondents perceived genetics knowledge as less important than other facets of professional practice (e.g., family dynamics), and they overwhelmingly endorsed the idea of mandatory course requirements in genetics as a requirement for a nursing degree and expressed a willingness to take such courses.

Nurses were also questioned on their confidence in discussing genetic information with patients. Nurses reported the highest level of confidence for standard practices such as taking a family history, and the least confidence with handling the particulars of genetic testing. "Nurses were less confident talking about genetics with patients," said Scanlon. "For example, they were most uncomfortable about explaining the implications of specific genetic tests."

More than 50% of nurses are sometimes involved with providing genetic services. This includes taking a family history of genetic disease or recording genetic information. However, nurses reported that they provided genetic information to patients only infrequently. Less than 40% of the nurses said they received requests for genetic information, but half of these refer the requests to someone else.

Nurses were also questioned on their attitudes toward ethical dilemmas that might arise during the course of providing genetic services. Half of the respondents said that spouses, adult siblings, and adult children of patients who submit to genetic tests have a right to share in test results. Seventy-five percent thought employers, schools, government, and insurance companies had no right to access genetic information.

"Twenty-two percent of the nurses thought that genetic information should be held to a higher standard of privacy, but seventy-five percent thought it should be treated as other health information," said Scanlon. "Ninety percent of the nurses felt that parents with genetic conditions should alert children to the presence of a family history."

The most controversial ethical dilemmas related to reproductive decisions. "Nurses were split over whether parents have a duty not to bring a child into the world with genetic disease," says Scanlon. "And the majority disagreed with the statement that it is unethical to test for genetic disease when there is no available treatment."

The survey highlighted the fact that nurses need more resources to help them recognize the importance of genetics in health care and to help them adequately respond to present and future requests for genetic services. Scanlon says the ANA is actively trying to develop resources for nurses. "We need both continuing education and curriculum development," says Scanlon.

Margaret Grey, of the Yale School of Nursing, reported on an informal survey she conducted of nursing colleagues at different schools throughout the country. She found similar results to those reported by ANA's Scanlon. Nursing faculty members polled at ten different schools reported that students are required to take undergraduate courses in biology and chemistry, but not in molecular biology. In addition, most nursing curricula involve 6–10 credit hours of basic science and pathology, and include some discussion of genetics. However, nursing faculty members at some schools reported instruction in the clinical implications of mutations in the cystic fibrosis transmembrane conductance regulator (CFTR) gene, which can cause cystic fibrosis. At the master's level, Grey's colleagues reported that nursing students typically receive 6–24 hours of lectures (not credit hours) in genetics.

"This suggests that there is a huge continuing education need," says Grey. Nurses typically do not have a strong background in molecular biology and genetics to interpret all the research in these fields, she says. "But how will we get there? How do we hook providers? We can't refer everyone to a genetic specialist."

Grey says that because nursing curricula are relatively fluid and amenable to change, new information in medical genetics can be integrated into programs rather quickly. "Our biggest challenge is not for the new practitioner," she says. "We will have to come up with creative ways to get those now practicing up to speed." Grey suggests that computers and networks have great potential for filling the knowledge gap among practicing nurses. "Computers can be useful, because people won't be embarrassed to ask basic questions."

Grey says it is important to turn to the nursing community to help deliver genetics information. "The essence of nursing is the ability to deal with clients at their level," says Grey. "Nurses have the ability to help get clients to where they need to be. Not many senior scientists have developed strength in this area."

PHYSICIANS: GENETICS KNOWLEDGE AND ATTITUDES

As genetics discoveries continue to be made, more and more genetics services will be provided by primary care providers, who usually serve as the introduction to the health care system for patients at risk for genetic disease, according to Neil Holtzman of Johns Hopkins University in Baltimore. "We felt it was important to get a baseline knowledge assessment of these physicians as well as an understanding of their attitudes toward delivering genetic service," said Holtzman at the first Banbury meeting. "We prepared a questionnaire of 26 questions whose main thrust was to determine what primary care physicians knew about genetics." Questions included information on basic Mendelian genetics, definitions of genetic terms, and calculations of genetic risk and probability.

Interestingly, in a pilot study of their survey, Holtzman and colleagues found that only 20% of the physicians responded. However, when the researchers offered physicians $25 to complete the survey, 65% completed the questionnaire. In contrast, 80% of medical geneticists and genetic counselors responded to the questionnaire in the absence of financial incentives.

In all, 1140 primary care physicians and psychiatrists returned questionnaires designed to assess their knowledge of medical genetics. Overall, the study population averaged a 73% score for correct responses. The highest scores were found among genetic counselors and medical geneticists, followed by pediatricians.

Not surprisingly, those who had greater exposure to genetics in their practice also performed better. "We separated respondents to the survey based on their exposure to genetics in their practice," said Holtzman. "We saw very significant differences in knowledge between high and low exposure specialties as well as differences based on the year of graduation from medical school. More recent graduates tended to score better."

The survey results were not explained by whether physicians had ever had a course in genetics, which did not seem to affect overall scores. "The most important factor seems to be whether the practitioner is exposed to genetics in practice," said Holtzman. "We shouldn't give up on physicians. When confronted with problems, they can learn very quickly."

Holtzman says the study may indicate that continuing education efforts should focus on the needs of the practitioner. "As long as continuing education is geared to their needs and as long as it's something that they want to learn and they perceive a need, the education efforts will be successful. To impose it on them will not do much better than a class in genetics in college or medical school."

William Freeman, of the American Academy of Family Physicians, is a family practitioner in Albuquerque, New Mexico. He agrees with Holtzman and says that educational efforts targeted toward physicians should take advantage of "teachable moments."

"Family physicians do want to learn to use tests well," said Freeman at the Banbury meeting. "We want to learn what medical genetics people can do for our patients. We want to learn what beliefs, cues, culture, and concerns affect patients' decisions. We want to know how to maximize the benefit and minimize the risks." Freeman says that physicians will learn when they need the information.

"How do we learn? Teachable moments," he says. "Teaching has to be brief, dispensed in practical units using multimedia, and delivered multiple times."

Fred McCurdy of the University of Nebraska cites several issues, needs, and barriers that must be considered in ensuring that physicians receive adequate training and education in genetics.

Issues:

- Genetics should be a prerequisite for medical school. The volume of information presented in medical school is so huge that faculty will resist adding more requirements to existing curricula.

- Use of diversity in carving out time in medical school curricula. Geneticists may have to carve out a niche in existing curricula. For example, at Nebraska, genetics was eased into the curricula as a self-directed learning component in pediatrics.

- The field is changing rapidly, and mechanisms must be developed for updating information in a timely manner. Information presented during the first year of medical school may be out of date by the fourth year.

- Turf battles among faculty members must be negotiated. The question of who teaches what aspects of new curricular components must be arrived at by consensus.

- Currently, there is a lack of a national coordination to invest in genetics education.

Needs:

- In genetics, as in other areas of instruction, students need to learn to apply principles from medical school to practical settings.

- Everyone needs to know genetics. In addition to MDs, nurses, pharmacists, dentists, and other health professionals must be educated.

- Physicians need to develop the use of information technology. In genetics, there is a great need for information on-line. Physicians don't want to appear uninformed and tend not to want to interact face to face.

Barriers:

- Turf issues. Physicians, genetic counselors, and nurses do not always agree on who should provide specific genetic services.

- Silo mentality. In medical school as well as medicine as a whole, there is a lack of interaction with other doctors and health care professionals.

- Lack of people to teach genetics and to deliver genetic services in medicine.

Training Models

Continuing Education for Nurses

Anne Matthews and her colleagues at the University of Colorado in Denver have developed a successful program aimed at disseminating genetic information to nurses and other health professionals through continuing education. The program, which was developed through the school of nursing in collaboration with the departments of medicine and genetics at the university, targeted nurses with roles as public health school nurses, nurse practitioners, OB-GYN nurses, high-risk nursery care providers, as well as physicians' assistants, social workers, and people who work with individuals with developmental disabilities.

"We first conducted a needs assessment survey to determine what would be helpful in the curriculum," said Matthews at the Banbury meeting. "We wanted to do something that could be taught in home communities that would provide nurses with a base for understanding genetic problems."

The goals of the program included:

- incorporating genetic information into nursing practice

- identifying patients with genetic disease or genetic conditions

- helping families use resources available to them

The Colorado curriculum was packaged in several units, each of which was accompanied by detailed lesson plans. Facilitators and teachers attended a one-week training program in Denver. Topics covered range from basic genetics to the impact of genetics on the family, and disease management. The curriculum also relies on video segments, computer-assisted tutorials, and discussions of ethical and legal issues.

"Class assignments include taking a pedigree from a client and conducting a case study in which students interview a family with a genetic disorder from their own caseload," says Matthews. "However, the course is not intended to train nurses to become geneticists or genetic counselors."

Matthews says that the Colorado curriculum has been used by 1800 professionals in 18 states. An impact study conducted several years ago indicated that nurses who had taken the course were more cognizant of genetic issues and made an effort to address these issues. As a result, she has observed an increase in referrals from people who have taken the course. The success of the course, says Matthews, is partly due to an attempt to seek input from the community and also to make it available on a local basis. In addition, the breakdown of the course into digestible units with complete lesson plans and supplementary materials has facilitated its widespread use. "The fact that nurses could take the course locally and that they could get credit for it was an attracting feature," says Matthews. "Also there was an awareness from lay literature that this was an area where patients were asking questions, particularly in the area of prenatal diagnosis." Matthews says that the curriculum is now being updated for future distribution.

Educating Primary Care Physicians

MEDICAL SCHOOL CURRICULA

Although many medical schools may be slow to change curricula, trends are changing at some schools, according to Myron Genel at Yale University. "I think there is a good deal of ferment in medical school curricula," he says. "The means exist to reform. One size does not fit all 126 schools or 126 curricula." Traditionally, medical school training has involved preclinical course work during the first two years and clinical training during the last two years. However, this trend is beginning to disappear, according to Genel. Yale, for example, has recently introduced a new initiative. During the first two years genetics and molecular biology are emphasized as part of the basic science training. During the fourth year, after students have received clinical training, basic science concepts are re-examined in a 4-week course.

"We attempt to bring basic sciences back to the clinic, to cement the relationship, in this 4-week course," says Tom Duffy, also of Yale. "During this period students will brainstorm on all aspects of cases involving hypertension, asthma, sickle cell anemia, and breast cancer. Part of this involves investigating the role of genetics and discussing the ethical implications. We hope that through this, students will be forced to bring basic science, including genetics, to the clinical experience."

Duffy and Genel say that attempts by medical schools to integrate clinical and basic science training and to develop interdisciplinary approaches to learning may create a window of opportunity to also integrate genetics education into the curricula. However, as with nursing, Genel says that the biggest hurdle will be keeping practicing physicians up to date on advances in medical genetics. "Continuing medical education will be our greatest challenge," says Genel. "The user has to want the information."

Continuing Education: A Regional Approach

One method for educating professionals in genetics, suggested by several participants at the Banbury meeting, involves enhancing opportunities in continuing education. Mary Esther Carlin, a medical geneticist in the Tarrant County Hospital District in Fort Worth, Texas, in conjunction with the Texas Genetics Network and the Texas Medical Association, has organized several symposia for local physicians in Fort Worth.

Seventy-two health care providers attended the first meeting orchestrated by Carlin—a 2-day symposium held in August, 1993. Of the attendees, half were physicians, 7 were speech pathologists, and 29 were nurses, students, or other health care professionals. At a second meeting, held in McAllen, Texas, where incidence of neural tube defect is high, attendance doubled. "It can make a difference, when you tailor the topics to the interests of the audience," says Carlin. "There is a lot of interest in neural tube defects in this region of Texas. In designing the program, we included talks centered on this topic. In addition, we involved the local community in the planning of the meeting and we encouraged their attendance."

Carlin offers several suggestions to enhance the success of continuing education efforts:

- Focus on timely topics of interest to the local lay and professional communities

- Feature local speakers and involve the local community

- Offer credit for continuing medical education

- Include minorities and offer bilingual public sessions

- Include private practitioners in addition to university-affiliated professionals

- Include a variety of medical disciplines

- Ask for suggestions from medical and lay community

Maternal and Child Health Initiatives

Jane Lin-Fu, Chief of the Genetics Services Branch, Maternal and Child Health Bureau of the Health Resources and Services Administration, Health and Human Services, in Rockville, Maryland, oversees the development of several government-initiated programs for genetic services. The mission of the Maternal and Child Health Bureau is to improve the health of all mothers and children. Although the bureau can develop programs that enhance the delivery of genetic services and the education of health care professionals, all programs must ultimately be funded by Congress. "We work with a very meager budget," says Lin-Fu. "The challenge is in determining how best to use it."

A major thrust of the maternal and child health bureau is strengthening the implementation of genetics in primary care, says Lin-Fu. This includes comprehensive care for patients and families affected by Cooley's anemia, sickle cell anemia, and thalassemia. In addition, the agency works at overcoming ethnocultural barriers, and in easing the transition from pediatric to adult care for individuals with genetic disorders.

The Genetics Services Branch funds nine special projects of regional and national significance (SPRANS) which are designed to educate primary care physicians. Among the other initiatives supported by the maternal and child health bureau are ten regional genetic networks, under the umbrella of the Council of Regional Networks for Genetic Services (CORN) and the Alliance of Genetic Support Groups, a consumer coalition. CORN brings together representatives from regional networks to encourage communication and planning for genetic services in addition to addressing national public health priorities.

Genetic Counselors' Initiatives

Karen Greendale, a geneticist with the New York State Department of Health in Albany, acknowledges that a shortage of genetic counselors exists. One approach, she says, to alleviating the need for genetic services is to involve genetic counselors in the training of other health professionals. "There are advantages to using genetic counselors to train other health professionals," says Greendale. "We have been trained in multiple disciplines, we have a psychosocial orientation, and we're available at low cost. The disadvantage is that we are not being trained to educate."

Funded by a grant from the Human Genome Project, Beth Fine of Northwestern University and her coworkers have developed a core curriculum to be used for training genetic counselors to educate other health care professionals in genetics. The Northwestern researchers have developed curricular materials and have trained 20 genetic counselors to teach the course to other health care professionals.

"The idea is to train health care workers to independently handle routine cases," said Greendale at the meeting, on behalf of Fine. "We hope to determine whether a short course can adequately prepare professionals. Can a little knowledge be a dangerous thing? Will they handle cases inappropriately if they are not appropriately trained?"

Professional Outreach

Jessica Davis, a physician and medical geneticist at Cornell University Medical College, has had success in teaching genetics to primary care practitioners through outreach programs. Long Island has 3.6 million inhabitants, but only 3 practicing geneticists. Davis and her Cornell colleagues began visiting different clinics on the island on an outreach basis to provide training in medical genetics to primary care practitioners. The program has been successful, says Davis, because they have encouraged practitioners to take primary responsibility in designing appropriate curricula as well as assisting in the planning and implementation of the program.

In a parallel program, Davis and her colleagues have also visited high schools to teach the students about medical genetics. She notes that since the program began, an increasing number of Westinghouse science scholarship winners come from Long Island in schools that have participated in the program, and many students have gone on to become geneticists.

Davis and her Cornell colleagues also helped to develop the genetics program at the Chinatown Health Center, as discussed at the first meeting. There, they developed a curriculum and hands-on training model that involved everyone on the health center staff. Now, Davis and her colleagues are trying to introduce the program developed for Chinatown to 10 other community-based clinics throughout New York City.

Davis says that she and her colleagues have learned several lessons key to the success of outreach educational efforts. First to keep in mind, she says, is that any outreach effort is a collaboration and it is important to establish a dialogue among all those involved. It is also important to assess the needs of the community and direct any educational efforts to the needs of the community. Outreach programs should also be content-oriented and involve the sharing of information.

"We are evaluating the impact of our programs not only by measuring new information gained, but also by assessing the impact of our program on clinical practice parameters," says Davis. "Our programs are also geared to strengthen ties between local health care providers and their nearest neighbor genetics program."

Professional Organizations

Other avenues involve professional outreach programs through professional societies. Deborah Runkle of the American Academy for the Advancement of Sciences discussed her organization's efforts to reach members of various health professional societies. "We're looking at societies representing members who don't deal with genetics on a daily basis, but for whom genetics is important." said Runkle. "We are designing educational modules for members that they can use in a variety of situations." Runkle says the materials under development are targeted for professional education, graduate pro-grams, continuing education efforts, and opportunities for reaching prac-titioners at "teachable moments."

As a first step, Runkle and her collaborators are surveying society mem-berships to assess their educational needs. "The goal will be to make discrete modules available to health care professionals," she says. "This will allow dif-ferent people to take materials out as they wish. This is not the only way to accomplish this, but it draws on our greatest strength."

Goals for Genetics Education

The issues involved in incorporating genetics into nursing and medical school education are similar. The primary hurdle that meeting participants anticipate is enlisting the support and enthusiasm of existing faculty and practicing health care professionals. Undergraduates and medical students can be re-quired to receive training in genetics and are probably more interested in it as a current and relevant discipline. For those who received their training before the first gene was cloned, however, genetics can seem like a very foreign, ir-relevant—and often intimidating—discipline. The challenge, most seem to agree, will be to get medical and nursing faculty interested enough in genetics to want to teach it to medical students, and to get practicing nurses and physicians interested enough in genetics to want to learn more about it and integrate it into their practice.

"We need to create a receptive climate for genetics education," says Suzanne Feetham. "But how do you create an interest in learning a new field for people who are already too busy?"

After considering several models for training other health care profes-sionals in genetics, several key areas and common threads important in the success of such efforts were cited. These include:

- *Knowledge base.* Identify and develop a core genetics knowledge base for all primary care health professionals. This should include biological genetic content and competencies for all levels of education, and counseling skills for providers of genetic services.

- *Continuum of genetics education.* Recognize that genetics is a bridge dis-cipline that cuts across all aspects of training in medicine, nursing, and allied health professions. Set the stage for an integrated continuum of edu-cation in genetics from the undergraduate levels through postgraduate and continuing education efforts. Strong linkages between didactic and clinical education experiences should be developed.

- *Curricular changes.* Encourage academic centers to incorporate genetics knowledge into curricula for health care professionals. Enlist the support of faculty and administrators to determine how medical genetics fit into the total curricula. A "buy-in" by faculty is needed to generate interest and enthusiasm for genetics. Incentives to bring faculty up to speed in genetics should be developed. Identify innovators among faculty who will take the lead in integrating genetics into existing curricula. Survey all medical, nursing, and allied health schools to evaluate genetics curricula and to assess needs at all educational levels. Identify gaps in knowledge and address these.

- *Teachable moments.* Develop ways to take advantage of teachable moments and provide opportunities for on-the-job training. The most opportune time to teach professionals about genetics is when they need the information. Mechanisms for dispensing information when the practitioner needs it may be particularly efficient. Support the development of a national clearinghouse and other innovative technologies such as multimedia, satellite hookups, and telemedicine consulting resources for providing on-the-spot genetics information.

- *Continuing education.* Develop and utilize continuing education programs for rapidly disseminating genetics curricula to health professionals. Involve professionals from the local community in assessing needs, and in planning and implementing educational programs. Provide incentives for practicing professionals to be involved in genetics education and to incorporate genetics into practice. Make continuing education programs accessible at the local level. Develop curricula for continuing education in digestible self-contained units. Make use of audiovisual aids, computer-assisted tutorials, multimedia materials, and other tools to reinforce concepts.

- *Professional organizations.* Utilize the influence of professional organizations to move the agenda of genetics education for primary health care providers. Develop continuing medical education courses in conjunction with professional medical societies. Try to influence state licensing boards to include proficiency in genetics as a requirement for licensing. Collaborate with specialty organizations for inclusion of genetics content in certification examinations.

- *Role of geneticists and genetic counselors.* Involve genetic counselors in the training of other health care professionals.

Afterthoughts

The Banbury meetings on Incorporating Genetics into Primary Health Care took an important first step in laying out some issues that will likely arise as primary care practitioners and genetic specialists begin the massive effort to move genetic services into primary care practice. However, identifying problems and barriers and deciding what needs to be done doesn't necessarily mean the job is going to get done.

Meeting participants agreed that the discussion groups arrived at goals worth pursuing. "We need to ensure mechanisms to move these recommendations forward," said Jessica Davis. But how? It is unrealistic to expect one small gathering of health care professionals and policymakers to solve all the problems of genetics and health care, and some of the hurdles are not unique to genetics.

"Some of the issues, such as ensuring access to genetic services, are the same issues encountered in ensuring access to primary care," says Janet Heroux, of the Robert Wood Johnson Foundation. "This is a challenge the Robert Wood Johnson Foundation has been grappling with for more than 20 years. The barriers to genetics are similar to those encountered in primary care. There are financial, geographic, and cultural barriers to obtaining genetic services, just as there are in obtaining health care in general."

Most of the meeting attendees agreed that it will be important to develop model systems of care and that the best approach will be to fund demonstration projects. Funding for such proposals would be solicited through both private and federal funding organizations. However, the criteria for selecting for funding such proposals was a matter of discussion.

Although some participants believed that it is too early to develop models for delivery of genetics services and that more research is needed, others believed that now is the time to begin looking at how some practices are already incorporating genetics into primary care. There are several programs that address some of these primary care practice issues. However, in order to accomplish assimilation of genetic services into primary care, the dialogue between educators, practitioners, scientists, and policymakers must increase, and current programs must be strengthened.

"Is the notion of seeking models a good way to demonstrate how genetics can or should be incorporated into primary care?" said Holtzman. "If so, then what do those models have to address?"

Reed Pyeritz of the American College of Medical Genetics offered another view. "There is still much basic research that needs to do be done. I don't think we're ready to deliver models for genetic services."

William Freeman perhaps summed up the sentiments of the majority of those in attendance, and it is likely that future efforts stemming from the meeting will follow his suggestion. "There are many parameters that need to be measured in assessing the success of any model," he said. "Some things need to be measured, but we first have to develop the tools. This should be researched. But by default, there will already be systems out there. We may not have the luxury of developing everything in sequence."

Nancy Touchette

Further Reading

Burke, W., M. Daly, J. Garber et al. 1997. Recommendations for follow-up care of individuals with an inherited predisposition to breast cancer. II. BRCA1 and BRCA2. *JAMA* **277:** 997.

Forsman, I. 1988. Education of nurses in genetics. *Am. J. Hum. Genet.* **43:** 552.

Geller, G., E.S. Tambor, G.A. Chase, K.J. Hofman, R. Faden, and N.A. Holtzman. 1993. Incorporation of genetics in primary care practice. *Arch. Fam. Med.* **2:** 1119.

Hofman, K.J., E.S. Tambor, G.A. Chase, G. Geller, R.R. Faden, and N.A. Holtzman. 1993. Physicians' knowledge of genetics and genetic tests. *Acad. Med.* **68:** 625.

Holtzman, N.A. 1989. *Proceed with caution.* Johns Hopkins University Press, Baltimore, Maryland.

Lea, D.H., J.K. Williams, and S.T. Tinley. 1994. Nursing and genetic health care. *J. Gen. Couns.* **3:** 113.

Levitan, M. 1988. *Textbook of human genetics.* Oxford University Press, New York.

Marteau, T. and M. Richards. 1996. The troubled helix: Social and psychological implications of the new human genetics. Cambridge University Press.

Nelkin, D. and M.S. Lindee. 1995. *The DNA mystique.* W.H. Freeman and Company, New York.

Schneider, K.A.. 1994. *Counseling about cancer: Strategies for genetic counselors.* Graphic Illusions, Dennisport, Massachusetts.

Institute of Medicine. 1994. *Assessing genetic risk: Implications for health and social policy.* National Academy Press, Washington, D.C.

Scanlon, C.and W. Fibison. 1995. *Managing genetic information: Implications for nursing practice.* American Nurses Association, Washington, D.C.

Tambor, E.S., B.A. Bernhardt, G.A. Chase, R.R. Faden, G. Geller, K.J. Hofman, and N.A. Holtzman. 1994. Offering cystic fibrosis carrier screening to an HMO population: Factors associated with utilization. *Am. J. Hum. Genet.* **55:** 626.

Watson, J.D., M. Gilman, J. Witkowski, and M. Zoller. 1992. *Recombinant DNA* (2nd. Ed.). Scientific American Books, New York.

APPENDIX A

It's in the Genes

Inside each cell in the human body resides the hereditary material known as deoxyribonucleic acid (DNA). DNA combines with certain proteins to form the chromosomes. DNA is made up of a string, or chain, of small units known as nucleotides. The sequence of nucleotides along the strands of DNA within each cell determines, to a large extent, the unique genetic characteristics of the individual.

Within each chromosome and along the DNA strand reside the 100,000 or so genes that code for all the proteins a person needs to function as a human being. Sometimes, the DNA within the chromosomes can become damaged. If the damage is not repaired correctly, a mutation, or change in the DNA sequence, can occur. Usually mutations in DNA are of no consequence; however, if a mutation occurs in a gene that codes for a protein important for the function of a particular cell, cell function can be disrupted, and disease can occur.

Not all diseases due to genetic mutations are inherited. If mutations occur in the somatic cells of the body, they cannot be passed on to offspring. However, if mutations occur in the germline cells—eggs or sperm—the mutation can be passed on from generation to generation. Germ-line mutations can be especially severe because they can affect all the cells in the body.

The science of genetics deals with the patterns of inheritance of genes. Some genetic traits follow the simple inheritance patterns first described by Gregor Mendel, a monk who lived in the 1800s. Mendelian genetic traits can be autosomal dominant (they cause an effect even if only one mutated gene is inherited), autosomal recessive (they cause an effect, but only if two mutant genes are inherited, or X-linked (the defect lies on the X-chromosome and causes an effect primarily in males). If a gene mutation is dominant and carried by one parent, an individual stands a 50% chance of inheriting a mutant gene. If a gene is recessive, and both parents carry one normal and one mutant gene, a person stands a 25% chance of developing disease, a 50% chance of being a carrier, and a 25% chance of inheriting no mutant genes.

Not all genes follow such simple patterns of inheritance. Some mutated genes can be inherited, but show no effect unless other genes are also mutated or the individual is exposed to certain environmental factors. These genes have a lower "penetrance" than genes for Mendelian traits. Such is the case with many cancers, which develop only after several essential genes are mutated in a cell. Although individuals with a particular disease may carry mutations in a particular gene, not all people with mutations in the gene will necessarily develop the disease. Predicting the risk of developing a genetic disease in such a case is much more difficult than with Mendelian genes.

Today, research aimed at identifying mutations in many genes that can cause disease is progressing at a furious pace, due largely to the Human Genome Project. The Human Genome Project is a government-funded collaborative effort by laboratories throughout the United States and other countries to identify and sequence all the genes in the human genome. So far, approximately 2,000 genes have been mapped, or located, on the DNA strand. When mutated, 900 of these genes have been shown to cause disease.

As new genes are identified, researchers have set out to develop tests that can determine whether certain disease-causing mutations are present in an individual's genome. DNA-based tests promise to help geneticists, genetic counselors, and other health care professionals assess with greater certainty the risks of inheriting or developing genetic disease.

APPENDIX B

As genetic tests make their way into mainstream medicine, further complexities are likely to confuse both consumers and health care providers alike. As discussed by Francis Collins, allelic heterogeneity—hundreds of mutations within a single gene within the population that have the capacity to cause disease—and the effects of several different genes, some of which may be influenced by environmental factors, make it difficult to predict the risk of genetic disease. The situation gets even murkier when contemplating the effects of test sensitivity and specificity in predicting genetic disease through testing.

James Allen of the AMA presented data at the first meeting on how accurately genetic tests of varying sensitivity and specificity should be able to predict disease caused by genetic mutations of varying frequency within the population.

Table 1 illustrates how well a test would accurately predict the likelihood of genetic disease for a disease caused by a defect in a single gene. In this hypothetical case, the gene mutation, or defective, disease-causing gene has a frequency of 0.2, or appears in 20% of the population. Table 1A illustrates a test with a sensitivity of 0.9 (90% of patients with the disease will have positive tests) and a specificity of 0.95 (95% with no genetic mutation will test negative, but 5% will test positive). If 100,000 people are tested, one would expect 20,000 to have the defective gene. This test would detect 18,000 of those carrying the gene and would miss 2,000. No genetic mutation would be expected for 80,000 people. This test would pick up 76,000 people as testing negative. However, 4,000 people would test positive when they in fact have no genetic mutation. Therefore, the predictive value of positive test (PVP) is 0.818 (18,000/22,000) and the predictive value of a negative test (PVN) is 0.974.

As shown in Table 1, B and C, more sensitive and specific tests yield higher predictive values. For a test with a 99% sensitivity and 99% specificity, the positive predictive value will be 96.1% and the negative predictive value will be 99.7%. For tests with a sensitivity and specificity of 99.9%, the predictive value is even greater. (PVP = 99.6 and PVN = 99.97).

For tests that detect genes that occur at a lower frequency in the general population, however, the situation is less encouraging. Consider a hypothetical gene that occurs in 1% of the population, as shown in Table 2. If a test has a sensitivity of 90% and a specificity of 95%, then the predictive value of a negative test will be 99.9% and the predictive value of a positive test will only be 15.4%. That means that of all the test results that come back positive, only 15.4% will truly be positive—nearly 85% will be false positives.

As the test sensitivity and specificity increase, so too does the predictive value. For example, as the test sensitivity and specificity approach 100% (99.9%), the predictive value of a positive test is 91% and that of a negative test is 100%. However, tests designed to detect genetic mutations that occur infrequently in the general population may be of questionable value in predicting positive tests results, as shown in Tables 3 and 4. Even at high test specificity and sensitivity (99.9%), the predictive value of a positive test for a genetic mutation that occurs in 1 out of 1000 people is only 50%. For a gene mutation that occurs in 1 out of 10,000 people, the predictive value of a positive test is less than 10%.

Allen points out that many disease-causing genetic mutations occur at low frequencies in the general population. Most current genetic tests will pick up only a fraction of all of the possible mutations that can exist. Thus, even for diseases caused by a single mutation in a single gene, interpreting test results may be overwhelmingly complex. Whether primary care physicians and other health care professionals are prepared to deal with such complexities remains uncertain and is definitely an aspect that needs to be addressed, says Allen.

Table 1. Gene "A" frequency = 0.2

Test:		A. Test sensitivity = 0.90 Test specificity = 0.95 +	–	Total
Gene	yes	18,000	2,000	20,000
"A"	no	4,000	76,000	80,000
	total	22,000	78,000	100,000

PVP = 0.818
PVN = 0.974

Test:		B. Test sensitivity = 0.99 Test specificity = 0.99 +	–	Total
Gene	yes	19,800	200	20,000
"A"	no	800	79,200	80,000
	total	20,600	79,400	100,000

PVP = 0.961
PVN = 0.997

Test:		C. Test sensitivity = 0.999 Test specificity = 0.999 +	–	Total
Gene	yes	19,980	20	20,000
"A"	no	80	79,920	80,000
	total	20,060	79,940	100,000

PVP = 0.996
PVN = 0.9997

(PVP) Predictive value of a positive test; (PVN) predictive value of a negative test.

Table 2. Gene "B" frequency = 0.01

Test:		+	−	Total
		A. Test sensitivity = 0.90		
		Test specificity = 0.95		
Gene	yes	900	100	1,000
"B"	no	4,950	94,050	99,000
	total	5,850	94,150	100,000

PVP = 0.154
PVN = 0.999

Test:		+	−	Total
		B. Test sensitivity = 0.99		
		Test specificity = 0.99		
Gene	yes	990	10	1,000
"B"	no	990	98,010	99,000
	total	1,980	98,020	100,000

PVP = 0.500
PVN = 0.999

Test:		+	−	Total
		C. Test sensitivity = 0.999		
		Test specificity = 0.999		
Gene	yes	999	1	1,000
"B"	no	99	98,901	99,000
	total	1,098	98,902	100,000

PVP = 0.910
PVN = 1.000

(PVP) Predictive value of a positive test; (PVN) predictive value of a negative test.

Table 3. Gene "C" frequency 0.001

| | | A. Test sensitivity = 0.90 Test specificity = 0.95 | | |
Test:		+	−	Total
Gene	yes	90	10	100
"C"	no	4,995	94,905	99,900
	total	5,085	94,915	100,000

PVP = 0.018
PVN = 0.999

| | | B. Test sensitivity = 0.99 Test specificity = 0.99 | | |
Test:		+	−	Total
Gene	yes	99	1	100
"C"	no	999	98,901	99,900
	total	1,098	98,902	100,00

PVP = 0.090
PVN = 1.000

| | | C. Test sensitivity = 0.999 Test specificity = 0.999 | | |
Test:		+	−	Total
Gene	tes	100	0	100
"C"	no	100	99,800	99,900
	total	200	99,800	100,000

PVP = 0.500
PVN = 1.000

(PVP) Predictive value of a positive test; (PVN) predictive value of a negative test.

Table 4. Gene "D" frequency 0.0001

Test:		A. Test sensitivity = 0.90 Test specificity = 0.95		
		+	–	Total
Gene	yes	9	1	10
"D"	no	5,000	94,990	99,990
	total	5,009	94,991	99,990

PVP = 0.002
PVN = 1.000

Test:		B. Test sensitivity = 0.99 Test specificity = 0.99		
		+	–	Total
Gene	yes	10	0	10
"D"	no	1,000	98,990	99,990
	total	1,010	98,990	100,000

PVP = 0.010
PVN = 1.000

Test:		C. Test sensitivity = 0.999 Test specificity = 0.999		
		+	–	Total
Gene	yes	10	0	10
"D"	no	100	99,890	99,990
	total	110	99,890	100,000

PVP = 0.091
PVN = 1.000

(PVP) Predictive value of a positive test; (PVN) predictive value of a negative test.

Incorporating Genetics into Primary Care: Views of Leaders in Genetics, Medicine, and Nursing

In a recent report, the Institute of Medicine predicted that primary care will eventually include genetic testing services (Andrews et al. 1994). Primary care physicians and nurses may need to provide genetic counseling and testing for several reasons: Advances in genetics are increasing the number of conditions that can be detected through genetic testing; media coverage of these new tests is stimulating consumer demand for information and testing, but the supply of genetics professionals is widely predicted to be insufficient to adequately counsel these consumers. Informed consumers are likely to approach primary care providers first, whereas uninformed consumers who could benefit will need to be identified. However, few primary care providers have received formal training in genetics (Geller and Holtzman 1991; Holtzman 1992; Hofman et al. 1993; Andrews et al. 1994). As worldwide efforts to map and sequence the entire human genome proceed, the need for primary care providers trained in genetics will only increase.

In anticipation of this need, the Robert Wood Johnson Foundation sponsored two meetings of leaders in primary care, human genetics, and nursing and medical education. Prior to the second meeting, we conducted a mail survey of the invitees to acquaint them with some of the facts and issues to be discussed at the meeting, and also to determine their opinions regarding the role of primary care physicians and nurses in the provision of genetic testing services. Preliminary findings of the survey were presented at the meeting in order to facilitate a more informed discussion. The results reported here summarize the initial impressions and opinions of respondents regarding the future of genetics in primary care.

Methods

Survey Instrument

The survey instrument consisted of a mail questionnaire designed to solicit opinions about the provision of genetic testing services by primary care providers in general, as well as respondents' opinions about currently available and possible genetic test/disease scenarios (see Appendix). Factual information was presented, followed by questions about how interested in these tests respondents thought the general public would be, the appropriateness of directive counseling, and the importance of different types of genetic testing services in primary care. Opinions about the importance of possible barriers were also solicited. All of the opinion questions used a six-point Likert response scale. Finally, information on the professional characteristics of each respondent was obtained.

Analysis

We hypothesized that opinions would be related to professional characteristics such as recency of graduation from medical or nursing school and having a specialty in genetics, as well as features of the genetic test/disease scenarios, such as the availability of effective treatment. Although we sent the questionnaire to a convenience sample, we tested the hypotheses using paired t-tests for comparisons of scaled responses to different questions, and t-tests, analysis of variance (ANOVA), and Tukey's HSD test for comparisons between different demographic/professional groups. The associations between professional characteristics were tested using the chi-square test. Only comparisons that were significant at the $p<.05$ level are shown in the tables.

Results

Response Rate and Demographic Characteristics

The questionnaire was sent to all fifty-five invitees to the second conference. Thirty-five people completed and returned the questionnaire before the conference began, and one returned the questionnaire at the conference for a final response rate of 93.5% among those thirty-one who attended. Seven of those who did not attend (29.2%) completed the questionnaire and were included in the analyses (see Table 1).

Table 1 also presents the demographic/professional characteristics of the respondents. More than half had a medical degree and nearly half had at least one nursing degree. Most respondents with a medical degree received their highest degree before 1980 (90%), compared to only 28.6% of those with a nursing degree (chi-square, $p<.001$). The most common place of work was an academic or professional organization (50%), followed by government

Table 1. Characteristics of Respondents ($n = 36$)

	Number	Percent
Attended second conference		
yes	29	80.6
no	7	19.4
Degree		
nursing	16	44.4
M.D. or other doctorate	19	52.8
M.S. (genetic counseling)	1	2.8
Year of most advanced degree		
before 1980	22	62.9
1980 and after	13	37.1
Organization where most work is done		
health care	8	22.2
academic/professional	18	50.0
government/nonprofit	10	27.8
Medical or nursing specialty		
primary care or other	24	66.7
genetics	12	33.3

(27.8%) and health care settings (22.2%). One third of the respondents listed genetics as either their primary or secondary specialty, whereas the remainder were either in primary care specialties such as family medicine or other specialties.

Perceived Level of General Public Interest in Genetic Tests

Respondents were asked how interested they thought the general public would be in different genetic test/disease scenarios on a scale from 1 (very interested) to 6 (very uninterested). Newborn screening for treatable, early-onset diseases had a significantly higher perceived level of interest than carrier-screening and prenatal diagnosis for untreatable diseases (mean ± S.D. = 2.8 ± 1.3 vs. 2.1 ± 1.2; $p<.01$). Similarly, respondents perceived greater public interest in a test that detects 75% of mutations for a treatable single-gene disease than for an untreatable disease (mean = 2.4 ± 1.2 vs. 3.7 ± 1.2; $p<.001$). Geneticists (respondents who had a primary or secondary specialty in genetics) perceived a lower level of public interest than non-geneticists in a test that detects 75% of the mutations for a treatable disease (mean = 3.2 ± 1.5 vs. 2.0 ± .8; $p<.05$).

Importance and Appropriateness of Genetic Counseling

Table 2 shows the respondents' views about genetic counseling. Respondents thought it very important to provide genetic counseling to healthy people

Table 2. Importance of Genetic Counseling and Appropriateness of Directive Counseling in Specific Situations

Genetic test/disease	Mean	S.D.
Importance of counseling healthy people when offering:		
carrier testing for untreatable, single-gene diseases	1.5	0.8
test for risk of developing monitorable, untreatable,		
late onset disorder	1.6	1.0
Appropriateness of *telling* people whether to:		
have an asymptomatic test for untreatable diseases	4.7	1.7
geneticists	5.8	0.6
non-geneticists	4.2	1.9[d]
abort fetus with severe disease	5.3[a]	1.4
geneticists	5.9	0.3
non-geneticists	5.0	1.7[e]
have test for treatable diseases	3.7[b,c]	2.2
most advanced degree obtained before 1980	3.1	2.1
most advanced degree obtained after 1980	4.7	2.1[e]
geneticists	4.8	1.8
non-geneticists	3.1	2.2[e]

Importance scale ranged from 1 (very important) to 6 (very unimportant). Appropriateness scale ranged from 1 (very appropriate) to 6 (very inappropriate).

[a]T, $p<.05$ compared to "have an asymptomatic test for untreatable diseases."
[b]T, $p<.001$ compared to "have an asymptomatic test for untreatable diseases."
[c]T, $p<.001$ compared to "abort fetus with severe disease."
[d]T, $p<.01$.
[e]T, $p<.05$.

who are offered either carrier testing for untreatable single-gene diseases or testing for risk of developing untreatable diseases. Most respondents thought that directive counseling is very inappropriate, except when counseling about the decision to have a test for a treatable disease.

Views on directive counseling significantly differed by specialty for all three scenarios and by year of most advanced degree for only one. Geneticists thought directive counseling was less appropriate than did non-geneticists. Respondents who obtained their most advanced degree in 1980 and after thought directiveness was less appropriate compared to those whose advanced degree was before 1980. There was no confounding between specialty and year of most advanced degree.

Incorporating Genetics into Primary Care

Respondents were asked for their opinions regarding the need for and the feasibility of incorporating genetics into primary care (scale ranged from 1 =

strongly agree to 6 = strongly disagree). Most agreed that genetic testing and counseling will soon be needed in primary care (mean = 1.8 ± .8). Most also agreed that it is feasible for these services to be part of primary care (mean = 2.1 ± 1.0).

Table 3 presents the perceived importance of offering different genetic services in primary care. Respondents thought all services were moderately important to provide in primary care, except management of patients with rare, single-gene disorders.

Table 3. Importance of Genetics in Primary Care

Question	Mean	S.D.
Importance of offering these services:		
population-based carrier screening	2.3	1.3
population-based screening for inherited susceptibility mutations	2.6	1.4
testing in high-risk families	2.1	1.3
genetic counseling	2.1	1.3
managing patients with rare, single-gene disorders	4.4	1.5
Importance of factors affecting ability of primary care *physicians* to provide genetic counseling:		
the time they have available	1.4	0.9
care providers	1.0	0.0
academics/professionals	1.2	0.5
government employees	2.0	1.4[a]
their knowledge of genetics	1.2	0.4
their opinion of what is best for patients	3.3	1.6
nurses	4.0	1.5
M.D. and/or Ph.D.	2.9	1.6[b]
care providers	1.9	1.0
academics/professionals	3.6	1.6
government employees	4.0	1.6[a]
the patient's knowledge of genetics	3.5	1.5
Importance of factors affecting ability of primary care *nurses* to provide genetic counseling:		
the time they have available	1.7	1.1
their knowledge of genetics	1.2	0.5
their opinion of what is best for patients	3.7	1.7
nurses	4.4	1.6
M.D. and/or Ph.D.	3.3	1.6[b]
the patient's knowledge of genetics	3.4	1.7

Importance scale ranged from 1 (very important) to 6 (very unimportant).
[a]F, $p < .05$.
[b]T, $p < .05$.

Table 3 also summarizes the importance that respondents attached to factors that may affect the ability of primary care physicians and nurses to provide genetic counseling. Overall, time and knowledge appear to be important factors. Providers' opinions of what is best for patients was not as important a factor for respondents with only a nursing degree compared to those with M.D. or Ph.D. degrees. Care providers and academics thought physicians' time and opinion of what is best for patients were more important factors compared to respondents who work for the government.

Overall, respondents were neutral about whether physicians (mean = 2.5 ± 1.3) or nurses (mean = 2.6 ± 1.4) were likely to learn sufficient genetics through continuing education programs, journals, or other activities to be able to counsel patients about specific tests (1 = very likely, 6 = very unlikely).

The final question was open-ended and asked respondents to list the three most important issues in incorporating genetics into primary care. The five most frequent responses were: provider knowledge of genetics (82.4%), costs or reimbursement (47.1%), time constraints (38.2%), discrimination or confidentiality issues (26.5%), and provider attitudes and beliefs about genetics (26.5%). Geneticists were significantly more likely than non-geneticists to list provider attitudes ($p<.05$). No other professional characteristics were significantly associated with the issues listed.

Discussion

This survey provides new information about the opinions of some of the leaders in primary care and genetics regarding the needs, priorities, and potential barriers for genetic testing services in primary care. We make no claims that our sample is representative of all leaders in these fields, since our method of selection of non-genetics professionals may bias our findings toward those with a greater interest in genetics.

As expected, the most consistent difference in opinion was between geneticists and other providers. The most consistent finding was that geneticists were more likely to believe directive counseling was inappropriate. Interestingly, they were also more likely to list provider attitudes as an important issue in the incorporation of genetics into primary care. Recency of medical training was only related to one question about directive counseling, but it has also been associated with increased knowledge of genetics and genetic testing (Kapur et al. 1983; Hofman et al. 1993) and willingness to provide genetic counseling about prenatal diagnosis (Geller et al. 1993).

Most respondents perceived high levels of general public interest for most types of genetic tests, an expected result given the focus of the meeting. Respondents thought the general public would be more interested in tests for treatable conditions, although few of these are yet available. Therefore, there may still be time to educate primary care providers before more acceptable tests become available.

Most respondents agreed that primary care providers could offer a range of genetic tests and genetic counseling. Offering genetic counseling was generally thought to be very important, although we confirmed previous findings that non-geneticist providers may not adhere as well to the principle of nondirectiveness as geneticists (Geller et al. 1993; Geller and Holtzman 1995). Respondents thought directiveness was more appropriate when counseling about testing for treatable conditions. We also found that more recent graduates were less directive, similar to findings of a study by Geller and others (Geller et al. 1993).

Perhaps the most valuable information gained from this survey is the identification of barriers to incorporating genetics into primary care by some of the leaders in the field. The three most frequently cited barriers were knowledge, financial, and time constraints, similar to a recent in-depth study of non-geneticist physicians (Geller and Holtzman 1995). Non-geneticist physicians were not confident about their knowledge of, or ability to discuss, genetic tests. This was especially true for tests for risk of developing a disease, although they thought their confidence would improve with more experience and exposure. Among those who did feel confident, they felt that the limited time they could spend with a patient would inhibit their ability to offer genetic counseling.

These results underscore the importance of educating primary care providers about genetic counseling, which remains the greatest challenge to incorporating genetics into primary care practice. Respondents were not in agreement about whether primary care physicians or nurses could learn sufficient genetics through continuing education and other activities to provide adequate genetic counseling. The success of alternative strategies for incorporating genetics into primary care education and practice needs to be assessed in order to more effectively train primary care providers to help deliver genetic testing services.

Teresa Doksum
Neil A. Holtzman

References

Andrews, L.B., J.E. Fullarton, N.A. Holtzman, and A.G. Motulsky, eds. 1994. *Assessing genetic risks: Implications for health and social policy*. National Academy Press, Washington, D.C.

Geller, G. and N.A. Holtzman. 1991. Implications of the human genome initiative for the primary care physician. *Bioethics* **5**: 318–325.

———. 1995. A qualitative assessment of primary care physicians' perceptions about the ethical and social implications of offering genetic testing. *Qualitative Health Research* **5**: 97–116.

Hofman, K.J., E.S. Tambor, G.A. Chase, G. Geller, R.R. Faden, and N.A. Holtzman. 1993. Physicians' knowledge of genetics and genetic tests. *Academic Medicine* **68(8)**: 625–632.

Holtzman, N.A. 1992. The diffusion of new genetic tests for predicting disease. *FASEB J.* **6**: 2806–2812.

Kapur, S., J.V. Higgins, A. Doughty, and D.J. Kallen. 1983. Medical practice and genetics in the mid-Michigan area. *J. Med. Educ.* **58**: 186–198.

APPENDIX

Survey Instrument

Incorporating Genetics into Primary Care: The Role of Physicians and Nurses

APPENDIX: SURVEY INSTRUMENT
Incorporating Genetics into Primary Care: The Role of Physicians and Nurses

Name: _____

Telephone: _____ Fax: _____ email: _____

1. Circle all degrees you hold:

   B.A.   B.S.   B.S.N.   M.A.   M.S.   M.S.N.   M.D.   Ph.D.   R.N.   Other _____

2. Year in which you obtained your most advanced degree (circle one)

   Before 1960   1960-69   1970-79   1980-89   1990-

3. Place a **1** in front of the activity that best characterizes your most important professional activity and a **2** in front of your next most important activity, if you have more than one.

   ___ Administrator   ___ Researcher

   ___ Educator   ___ Other: _____

   ___ Practitioner

4. Where do you do most of your work (check one)

   ___ Ambulatory care site other than managed care (e.g., private office)

   ___ Government agency

   ___ Hospital   ___ School of medicine

   ___ Managed care site (HMO, etc.)   ___ School of nursing

   ___ Professional organization   ___ Other: _____

5. Place a **1** in front of your primary medical or nursing specialty and a **2** in front of your secondary specialty, if you have one

   ___ Family practice   ___ Obstetrics/midwifery

   ___ Genetics   ___ Pediatrics

   ___ Internal medicine   ___ Other: _____

I.   Single-gene (Mendelian) diseases

The Human Genome Project is accelerating the discovery of genes for rare, single-gene (Mendelian) disorders (e.g., cystic fibrosis, Huntington disease, muscular dystrophy). The first step in the discovery of a gene is mapping it to a specific chromosome. When a gene has been mapped, linkage tests may be able to predict with high probability who will get the disease in families in which the disease has already occurred. The next step is identifying the gene and at least part of its DNA sequence. Neither of these steps requires knowing anything about gene function. The gene's role in disease causation is proven by showing that in people with the disease the gene has a different DNA sequence than in people without the disease. (Each unique sequence of a gene is called an <u>allele</u>.) Differences between alleles may be as small as one nucleotide, the unit of which DNA is composed. Such differences occur as a result of mutations in ova or sperm, which are then inherited.

Once a gene has been identified, tests to detect the presence of mutations can be readily developed and used in people regardless of whether they have a family history of the disease. This is genetic screening. However, until more is learned about normal function of the particular gene, no interventions to prevent or treat the disease in people born with a disease-causing genotype will, as a rule, be available. In this interim period (which may last for several years), people at risk of having affected children can avoid their conception by adoption or use of donor sperm or ova, or avoid their birth by prenatal diagnosis and abortion of affected fetuses.

6.   Imagine that a test has been developed that detects the mutations that are responsible for a rare, severely debilitating, single-gene disease that manifests early in life and shortens survival. The incidence of this disease is about 1 in 10,000, approximately that of phenylketonuria (PKU). Unlike PKU, the disease is untreatable. The disorder is a recessive, which means that to be affected a child must inherit disease-causing alleles from both parents. The parents, who each have one disease-related and one normal allele, are carriers and are not affected. About 1 in 50 people will be carriers. The test could be used to detect healthy carriers and also for prenatal diagnosis. At this stage of discovery, when <u>no treatment</u>, is available, how interested do you think the public in general will be in a predictive test?   (Circle the one number that best characterizes your opinion):

Very interested					Very uninterested
1	2	3	4	5	6

7.   Within 5 years, it is likely that a test will be available that can simultaneously detect at least 20 different severe, Mendelian diseases, using just a small amount of blood (from a finger prick) or buccal mucosa scraping. <u>Assume none of the diseases is treatable</u>. Their combined incidence is greater than 1 in 1,000 and about 1 in 15 healthy people will be carriers for at least one of the diseases. How interested do you think the public in general will be in such a "multiplex" test.

Very interested					Very uninterested
1	2	3	4	5	6

Some time after a gene has been identified, its function will be established. This could lead to "conventional" therapy, such as reduction of a dietary constituent that becomes toxic due to an inherited enzyme defect (e.g., reducing phenylalanine in PKU), or removing a toxic substance that accumulates due to an inherited transport defect (e.g., reducing copper by chelating agents in Wilson disease). After the normal human gene has been isolated, it can be inserted into bacteria and used to produce large amounts of the normal gene product, such as growth hormone or anti-hemophilia factor, which could be used to replace the defective gene product in those who will get the Mendelian disease.

2

The isolated normal gene could also be inserted into a harmless virus which could be administered to people who will get the disease in order to prevent severe disease from developing. Such "gene therapy" experiments are getting started for a few diseases, but will not be available routinely for several years.

8.   If treatments were developed for one or more rare, severe, early-onset disorders, but they had to be started in newborns, before symptoms appeared, in order to be effective:

	Very interested					Very uninterested
a) How interested would the public be in newborn screening for the disorder(s)	1	2	3	4	5	6
b) How interested would the public be in screening for carriers and in offering prenatal diagnosis to couples at high risk?	1	2	3	4	5	6

9.   Many mutations in a gene can each result in a Mendelian disease. Instead of being able to detect all such mutations, even the most sophisticated tests may only be able to detect about 75% of them.

	Very interested					Very uninterested
a) How interested do you think the public will be in a test that detects about 75% of mutations for any single-gene disease that is <u>untreatable</u>?	1	2	3	4	5	6
b) How interested do you think the public will be in a test that detects about 75% of mutations for any single-gene disease that is <u>treatable</u>?	1	2	3	4	5	6

II. Common, complex disorders

Gene mapping and other techniques have led to the discovery of genes that are associated with common, adult-onset, complex disorders, e.g., Alzheimer disease, cancer, coronary artery disease, and diabetes. Tests are already available that detect the presence of inherited susceptibility mutations (ISMs), which increase the probability that the person tested will get such a disease. Because other genetic and environmental factors must also be present, a positive test result does not predict future disease with certainty. Finding that a person has a positive test result could permit more intensive monitoring for the first signs of disease, e.g., mammography in young women found to have ISMs for breast cancer, or colonoscopy in young men and women found by testing to have ISMs for colon cancer. For colon cancer, presymptomatic detection can lead to survival to an older age through earlier surgery. The effectiveness of prophylactic surgery or chemoprophylaxis in women with ISMs for breast cancer has not yet been established. There is no treatment of proven efficacy that will prolong survival in patients with Alzheimers who have an associated genetic variant (apoE4). If insurance companies or employers become aware that an individual tests positive for an ISM for an untreatable disorder they may legally discriminate against them in most states.

10. ISMs in a gene will usually be found in 5 % or less of people who are eventually going to get a common disorder, like breast or colon cancer, or coronary artery disease. In most of the remaining 95%, environmental and multiple genetic factors will account for disease. If there is no proven means of improving survival in people with positive test results, how interested will the <u>general public</u> be in tests for ISMs for common disorders?

	Very interested					Very uninterested
	1	2	3	4	5	6

11. When a therapy is proven to be efficacious, compared to interest previously, do you think public interest in testing will be (circle one)

Very much greater	somewhat greater	slightly greater	not at all greater
1	2	3	4

Most, but not all, of the 5% of ISMs will be found in people who have more than one relative in which the disease has already occurred ("high risk families"). When an ISM is found in an asymptomatic relative in a high risk family, the chance that disease will occur is often between 50% and 90% in a normal lifetime.

12. Assume that presymptomatic monitoring in those with positive tests can detect disease early but that none of the surgical or medical treatments that are available have yet been proven effective. However, in families in which a particular ISM has been found in those with the disease, the finding that a relative at risk does <u>not</u> have the ISM spares that person of intensive monitoring and anxiety about getting the disease. (Risk is reduced to that of the general public.) Prenatal detection of the ISM is possible. How interested will asymptomatic people at risk of disease in <u>high risk families</u> be in tests for ISMs?

	Very interested					Very uninterested
	1	2	3	4	5	6

III. Genetic counseling

Genetic counseling helps people who are considering testing understand the options available if the test result is positive, including reproductive options, early monitoring, and possible treatment. Counselors also communicate the chances that the test will be positive, the chance that the test will give a wrong result or cause other harm, and the possibility that third parties might use the information to discriminate if they had access to the result. When a positive result is obtained, the genetic counselor will discuss these issues again, discuss the risk to other relatives, and help the individual and family cope with the result.

13. How important do you think it is to counsel apparently healthy people when offering genetic testing to determine if they are carriers of alleles for severe, early onset, single-gene (Mendelian) diseases for which there are no effective treatments?

	Very important					Very unimportant
	1	2	3	4	5	6

14. How important do you think it is to counsel apparently healthy people when offering genetic testing to determine if they are at increased risk of developing a late onset disorder for which monitoring for early warning is available but for which no effective treatment has been demonstrated?

Very important					Very unimportant
1	2	3	4	5	6

			Very appropriate					Very inappropriate

15. When there are no effective treatments, do you think it is appropriate to <u>tell</u> people whether or not to have the test? 1 2 3 4 5 6

16. If a woman decides to have prenatal diagnosis and the fetus is found to be affected, how appropriate do you think it is to <u>tell</u> the woman whether to abort or continue the pregnancy. Assume the test is for a rare, Mendelian disorder for which there is no effective therapy, and which results in severe disease and early death? 1 2 3 4 5 6

17. If an effective treatment became available that prevented the manifestations of a genetic disease, how appropriate would it be for counselors to <u>tell</u> people to have the test? 1 2 3 4 5 6

IV. Genetics in primary care

If genetic testing was to become widespread, there will not be enough professionals specifically trained to provide genetic counseling to meet the demand. Other means of providing this service will be needed.
Please indicate how strongly you agree or disagree with the following statements:

			Strongly agree					Strongly disagree

18. There will soon be a need for genetic testing and counseling to be part of primary care. 1 2 3 4 5 6

19. It is feasible for genetic testing and counseling to be part of primary care. 1 2 3 4 5 6

20. People who will be interested in new genetic tests currently have primary care providers. 1 2 3 4 5 6

21. Primary care providers can do little more than refer people to specialists for genetic testing. 1 2 3 4 5 6

5

Please rank how important it would be for each of the following services to be offered by <u>primary care providers</u>:

	Very important					Very unimportant
22. Carrier screening (population-based) 1	2	3	4	5		6
23. Screening for ISMs (population-based)..............................1	2	3	4	5		6
24. Testing in high risk families 1	2	3	4	5		6
25. Genetic counseling...1	2	3	4	5		6
26. Primary responsibility for managing patients with rare, single gene disorders..1	2	3	4	5		6

27. How important are each of the following in affecting the ability of primary care <u>physicians</u> to provide genetic counseling?

	Very important				Very unimportant
The time they have available 1	2	3	4	5	6
Their knowledge of genetics..1	2	3	4	5	6
Their opinion of what is best for the patient.......................1	2	3	4	5	6
The patient's knowledge of genetics...................................1	2	3	4	5	6

28. How important are each of the following in affecting the ability of primary care <u>nurses</u> to provide genetic counseling?

	Very important				Very unimportant
The time they have available 1	2	3	4	5	6
Their knowledge of genetics..1	2	3	4	5	6
Their opinion of what is best for the patient.......................1	2	3	4	5	6
The patient's poor knowledge of genetics............................1	2	3	4	5	6

	Very likely					Very unlikely

29. How likely do you think it is that <u>physicians</u> could learn sufficient genetics to be able to counsel about specific tests through continuing education programs, journals or other activities? 1   2   3   4   5   6

30. How likely do you think it is that <u>nurses</u> could learn sufficient genetics to be able to counsel about specific tests through continuing education programs, journals or other activities? 1   2   3   4   5   6

31. Please list the 3 most important issues in incorporating genetics into primary care:

   1. _____

   2. _____

   3. _____

Thank you for answering these questions. Please return in the stamped envelope to:

   Dr. Neil A. Holtzman
   Genetics and Public Policy Studies
   550 N. Broadway, Suite 511
   Baltimore MD 21205

Afterword: The Impact of the Human Genome Project on Medical Practice

When I was in medical school in the 1970s, students were taught that genetic diseases consist of thousands of rare, inherited disorders. These diseases were described as clustering within families and were characterized by their modes of inheritance: autosomal recessive, autosomal dominant, and X-linked.

During the past 20 years, however, as science has learned to manipulate and analyze the structure of human DNA and has studied inheritance patterns of more diseases in families, our concept of genetics has broadened dramatically. Indeed, the genetics revolution has arrived. Today, hardly a week passes without the publication of a research paper identifying a gene implicated in human disease. In just a few years, the roster of cloned disease genes has grown substantially, including genes involved in cystic fibrosis, inherited breast and ovarian cancer, Alzheimer's disease, Huntington's disease, Marfan syndrome, inherited colon cancer, and heart disease.

Now genetics is becoming the central science of biomedicine because nearly all human disease, except physical injury, is influenced by heritable changes in the structure or function of DNA. Efforts to understand and treat disease processes at the DNA level are becoming the basis for a new type of "molecular" medicine. By going directly to the source of human illness, molecular medicine strategies will allow health care providers to customize prevention and treatment strategies based on the unique genetic constitution of an individual. These tactics will apply not only to classic, single-gene hereditary disorders, but increasingly to more common, multi-gene disorders, such as cancer, heart disease, diabetes, and psychiatric illness.

The molecular approach to understanding and treating disease has received a tremendous push from the Human Genome Project, the international research program to develop technologies that make finding genes easier, faster, and cheaper. These technologies include genetic maps of molecular markers placed at high resolution throughout the human genome, physical maps consisting of sets of contiguous, cloned DNA spanning the entirety of each human chromosome; computer methods for easy data storage, retrieval, and manipulation, and ultimately, the complete nucleotide sequence of the human genome.

Assessing the ethical and social impact of new capabilities to obtain genetic information from individuals is also an integral part of the Human Genome Project. Indeed, the Ethical, Legal, and Social Implications (ELSI) program is unique among technology programs in its mandate to consider and deal with these issues alongside the development of the technology.

Launched in 1990, the Human Genome Project is a 15-year initiative that will provide detailed information about the structure and characteristics of human DNA, giving us the basic blueprint of a human being. By the year 2005—and some are predicting a year or two sooner—it will be possible to access a public database and read the complete order of all 3 billion nucleotides in the human genome, represented by the four-letter chemical alphabet A, T, C, and G.

When the project began, we had established an ambitious plan to guide the research through these initial years. Today we have met or exceeded most of those goals—some ahead of time and all under budget.

For example, in 1994, an international consortium headed by the Genome Science and Technology Center in Iowa published a genetic map containing almost 6,000 markers spaced less than 1 million bases apart. The density of markers on this map is four- to sixfold greater than the goals set in 1990, and it was accomplished more than a year ahead of schedule.

The first five-year goal for physical mapping—developing overlapping sets of cloned DNA that each spanned at least 2 million bases of DNA—has been easily exceeded. Physical mapping provides cloned sets of overlapping pieces of DNA that span a region of a chromosome, or even a whole chromosome, and serve as a resource for investigators who wish to isolate a gene they have located in a particular region on a chromosome. Today, these so-called "contigs" are many times longer than the plan called for, ranging from 20 to 50 million DNA bases in length. More than 95% of the human genome is covered by overlapping DNA clone sets, each of which is at least 10 million bases long.

Using the sequence-tagged site (STS) system of markers, genome scientists have developed a physical map that currently contains over 20,000 markers, half the number needed to meet the goal. The goal of adding 30,000 STS markers to the physical map, one every 100,000 bases, will likely be met soon. This detailed STS map will allow a skilled researcher to pinpoint the exact location of any gene within 100,000 bases of an STS marker. A recent initiative by private industry, which aims to produce short sequences of DNA from genes, will likely speed the rate of STS marker development and provide a resource for adding tens of thousands of markers from actual genes to the physical map.

Having met or exceeded our original goals for mapping, we now turn our vision for the next phase of the Human Genome Project to the most challenging technological undertaking of all: determining the sequence of DNA bases in the entire 3 billion base-pair length of human DNA. Knowing the order of DNA bases tells an investigator where genes are located as well as what instructions are carried in a piece of DNA. This information is critical to understanding the function of genes and how they cause disease. To date, technology development for this work has been primarily carried out experimentally on the DNA of important model organisms. Researchers sequencing the genome of the roundworm have now amassed over 50 million bases of DNA from that organism (over half of the animal's genome). These investigators expect to complete the sequence of the roundworm genome by the end of 1998.

Thus far, technology development in sequencing DNA has aimed at reducing cost and increasing rate. Although cost has been lowered to that called for in the five-year plan (about $0.50 per base), the rate of sequencing is still slower than that needed to complete the human genome by the year 2005. The National Human Genome Research Institute is therefore increasing emphasis on technology development for DNA sequencing to increase the speed of sequencing using current gel-based technologies. The urgency of pushing these advances now is considerable. Every reduction in cost of 1 cent per base pair will save $30 million in the production phase of sequencing the entire human genome. We now support human DNA sequencing projects at six U.S. universities.

Medical Implications of Gene Discovery

Genetic linkage mapping, physical mapping, gene identification, and DNA sequencing together make up the basic steps of a gene-isolation technique known as positional cloning. Positional cloning allows a researcher to identify a gene in the human genome and clone it when very little is known about the function of the gene in disease or normal biological processes. So far, over 60 disease-linked genes have been isolated using the positional cloning technique. Using these powerful tools, an investigator can isolate such genes in a matter of weeks or months, whereas it used to take as long as a decade.

Many of these gene discoveries are chronicled in the popular press. Daily newspapers regularly report the isolation of genes, and *Time, Life, U.S. News and World Report,* and *Newsweek* all have run cover stories on the medical implications of gene discoveries; so has nearly every major newspaper and television news show in the world. The mass media are currently the major carrier of information about genetic medicine to the public. Some of the information is accurate and some of it isn't; but more and more, patients are bringing the magazine or the newspaper into the health care provider's office wanting to know if they are genetically prone to a given disease.

We know that every human being inherits at least four or five (maybe more) marginally functional or nonfunctional genes that predispose them to various conditions or diseases. This is not to say that human disease is written into our genes as a preordained fact of life. Rather, these irregular genes may convey an increased risk to those who inherit them. It is the lifelong interplay of genes, environment, and life-style that will determine if, when, and how these predispositions manifest themselves.

Soon, with the rapid identification of disease genes and their translation into powerful DNA-based medical technologies, we can begin to answer those questions. By providing a blood sample, healthy patients can choose to have their DNA analyzed for specific gene changes. If a well-characterized mutation is found, the patient will know that he or she is at higher-than-average risk for a given disease. In other cases, the risk may be lower than average. The test results will then allow health professionals to begin customizing their care to the individual health needs of the patient.

This will also raise new challenges. Although health professionals will have the technology at hand to identify altered genes, they will often have to wait for safe and effective therapies to treat the disorder. This time lag between diagnosis and treatment has raised questions about whether we are really ready to offer testing for disease-linked DNA alterations on a large scale. How will the information stored in our genes be used? Will easy access to genetic information lead to thousands of otherwise healthy Americans losing their health insurance or jobs? Just as importantly, who is and who isn't socially, emotionally, or financially prepared to cope with these predictions?

The technical ability to perform tests for DNA mutations, therefore, should not be confused with a mandate to offer them. Safeguards must be in place to ensure that these tests are used wisely, maximizing their potential benefits to patients and minimizing their potential risks. One of the most critical safeguards is the enactment of laws to protect all Americans from discrimination based on the information in their genes. A few states have enacted some form of protection against genetic discrimination in health insurance. Last August, the President signed the Kasselbaum-Kennedy bill into law, creating this first federal law to address genetic discrimination in health insurance. Significantly more movement, however, will be needed on the state and federal legislative fronts in the coming years.

Another critical safeguard will be the expansion of genetic services within our health care system to help guide patients through the testing process, allowing them to make informed decisions about genetic testing. Numerous research studies show that specialized pre- and post-test counseling is critical for individuals to understand the implications of a positive or negative test result. Yet, today, there are only 2000 genetic counselors in the United States. Genetic counseling will need to become part of the role of the primary health care provider; but how will these counselors be trained?

Since its inception in 1990, the National Human Genome Research Institute has reserved about 5% of its annual budget to evaluate the ethical, legal, and social implications emerging from research on the human genome. The research community has already begun to study the necessary considerations for offering responsible genetic testing. For example, we are starting to learn more about the complexities of DNA testing for disease-linked alterations in the CFTR gene associated with cystic fibrosis and the BRCA1 gene associated with breast and ovarian cancer.

Cystic Fibrosis

Cystic fibrosis (CF) is the most common recessive genetic disorder in people of Northern European ancestry. One in every 25 people whose families originate from that region of the world are carriers of an altered CFTR gene. If a couple, each with a single copy of a misspelled CFTR gene, have a child, there is a 25% chance the child will inherit two altered copies of the gene that gives rise to CF and will develop the disease. There is a 50% chance a child of this couple will carry one altered copy of the CFTR gene and be a healthy carrier. However, most babies born with CF, some 80%, are conceived by parents who have *no* family history of the disease.

In August 1989, several research groups—including my laboratory at the University of Michigan—collaborated to isolate the CFTR gene on chromosome 7. The gene produces a protein that helps transport chloride ions across cell membranes. We found that in 70% of individuals with CF, a string of three bases (called $\Delta F508$) was deleted within the gene, thereby knocking out a single amino acid from the CFTR protein and making it nonfunctional. This supported the data cell biologists had generated previously about CF. In CF patients, the ability to transport chloride ions across cell membranes is greatly diminished. This leads to problems in the lungs and other physiological systems. Since the discovery of the CFTR gene, researchers have quickly developed a better understanding of the basic cellular defect involved in the disease, setting the stage for an intensive effort to bring drug and gene therapies into reality for CF.

Those are long-term efforts. The most immediate clinical impact of the gene's discovery has been CF carrier testing. Before finding the CFTR gene, genetic testing for the disease was available only to families with affected children and their close relatives. With the gene, it became possible for the first time to test any person for the $\Delta F508$ mutation. As we predicted in the paper announcing the isolation of the gene, it would thus be possible by DNA analysis to accurately diagnose nearly half of CF patients without a previous family history. Moreover, nearly 70% of those in the general population carrying one altered copy of the CFTR gene could be identified through genetic testing for the single, common $\Delta F508$ mutation.

Although the discovery of a single mutation seemed straightforward enough, the issues involved in CF testing have become increasingly complex.

Since finding ΔF508, researchers have identified over 600 possible misspellings in the CTFR gene. With so many alterations, it is not possible to look at one spot on the gene and predict a person's risk for CF. The situation is further complicated because some mutations may actually be benign variants. To compound the situation, some of these normally benign misspellings may indeed trigger disease in combination with other benign mutations.

This range of misspellings in the CFTR gene makes genetic testing for CF more technologically challenging. If one screens for the 6 most common mutations in the gene, genetic testing detects about 90% of all CF carriers of Northern European descent. This means one in six of all carriers will be missed.

All of these variables raise questions about the appropriate application of CF testing to medical practice. One question is, At what time is it most appropriate to test? A 1990 National Institutes of Health workshop on population screening for mutations in the CFTR gene suggested that ideally, prospective parents should be screened *before* they conceive to determine if they are carriers of a misspelled CFTR gene. A recent NIH Consensus Development Conference recommended that genetic testing for CFTR mutations be offered to all pregnant couples and those planning pregnancy, as well as those with a family history of the disease.

CF testing remains debated within the medical community, and studies show the general public harbors many misconceptions about genetic testing for CF carrier status. One problem is a lack of awareness about CF within the general population. Many people have never heard of CF or have inaccurate impressions of the disease. If individuals are not aware of CF, they will not be motivated to seek testing. If they are not educated about the disease, they cannot make a truly informed choice about whether to be tested.

Hereditary Breast Cancer

Genetic testing for CFTR alterations brings up issues important mainly to couples planning families, but testing for alterations in the BRCA1 gene, the major gene involved in hereditary, early-onset breast cancer, presents a different set of concerns: (1) The test predicts a level of risk for a disease that occurs in adulthood, and (2) we do not yet know the appropriate medical interventions for women whose disease is attributed to mutations in the BRCA1 gene.

About 5–10% of the 180,000 new cases of breast cancer reported annually in the United States occur in women with a strong family history of the disease. It has long been suspected that this familial predisposition could be traced to a specific gene or group of genes. In 1990, a region on chromosome 17 was shown to have a substantial role in early-onset familial breast and ovarian cancer. An intense hunt for the gene ensued, which culminated in

September 1994 with the isolation of the BRCA1 gene, the first major gene implicated in breast cancer.

In studies with approximately 200 families in which at least four closely related members had breast cancer, about half of the cases were attributed to BRCA1. This estimate rises to 75% in families with both breast and ovarian cancer. In many of these families, women who inherit an altered BRCA1 gene have a lifetime risk of breast cancer estimated to be as high as 85%. Approximately 400,000 women in the United States carry a BRCA1 mutation, but not all will develop breast cancer. Should we try to identify all of them?

BRCA1 is a large gene that spans 100,000 bases. Misspellings in the gene can occur anywhere. In fact, the current list of possible mutations in the gene has topped 100, including a number of apparently benign misspellings, or polymorphisms. With so many misspellings, the entire gene would need to be scanned for the presence of every possible mutation. It currently takes a research laboratory a couple of weeks to scan just one DNA sample, and at relatively high cost. Clearly, this approach is not yet feasible for routine testing of large numbers of women.

Another problem is that we cannot yet accurately determine the risk of breast cancer associated with each of the 100 or so BRCA1 mutations. Is it possible that a woman with a misspelling at point 1242 on the gene is at less risk for breast cancer than someone with a change at point 7421? Without this information, BRCA1 testing will lack the specificity for a precise interpretation of test results.

Assuming a BRCA1 mutation is found, we are still profoundly uncertain about the appropriate medical care of women with these mutations. Despite the general usefulness of mammograms for the early detection of breast cancer in women over the age of 50, there are no data to show that regular mammography at a younger age, in concert with self-examination and examination by doctors or nurses, will reduce the risk of death from metastatic breast cancer among very high-risk women with BRCA1 mutations.

We do not yet know the value of more drastic options, such as prophylactic mastectomy, in preventing breast cancer in these women, especially given the anecdotal evidence that cancer can still occasionally arise in the small amount of epithelial tissue remaining after surgery. There are no measures of proven value for the early detection of ovarian cancer in this particular group, and given occasional reports of peritoneal ovarian cancer years after prophylactic ovarian surgery, the quantitative effectiveness of the surgical approach in reducing the risk of ovarian cancer must be considered uncertain. It is possible that cancer should be treated differently in women with germ-line BRCA1 mutations, but at present there are insufficient data to guide the oncologist or surgeon.

Women from families with an identified BRCA1 mutation will usually benefit from being found not to carry the alteration, but women who test positive face a lifetime of potential consequences, such as discrimination in health insurance or jobs, or even in their personal lives, and uncertainty about their future health. Perhaps Sophocles was right when he said, "It is but sorrow to be wise when wisdom profits not."

Moreover, women who test negative must understand that they still face the same baseline 12% lifetime risk of breast cancer that any other woman faces. Extensive education and genetic counseling are thus needed for women who undergo such testing.

Given the many complexities involved in genetic testing for breast cancer predisposition, the American Society of Human Genetics, the National Breast Cancer Coalition, and the National Advisory Council of the National Center for Human Genome Research have emphasized the need for BRCA1 testing to remain a research activity for the time being.

Public Opinions about Genetic Testing

As genetic medicine becomes increasingly prominent in the news, Americans are developing attitudes about the subject based on the fragments of information they gather. In a 1992 survey by Louis Harris, 79% of respondents said they would take a genetic test, before having children, to find out the risk of having a child with a fatal disease. Some 64% said they would have a genetic test during pregnancy to determine whether the fetus had a genetic disease. Despite the prevalence of positive opinions about taking genetic tests, 68% of the people in this same study said they knew "relatively little" or "almost nothing" about genetic testing.

This survey capsulizes the challenges at hand for health care providers who will be confronted by increasing demands for genetic tests. Genetic tests in many cases may need to be thought of in the same way as new drugs being introduced into medical practice. Although they offer benefits to patients, genetic tests may also carry some risks or "toxicities" that need to be identified and understood so they can be minimized in the delivery of this growing health care technology.

Francis S. Collins

Index

A

Adult-onset diseases, genetic testing and, 22, 40
AIDS testing, 22
Allele, definition, 81
Alliance of Genetic Support Groups, 25
Alpha-fetoprotein analysis, 37
Alzheimer's disease, 8, 82, 87
    apolipoprotein e4 as risk factor, 7, 82
    chance of developing disease, family history and apolipoprotein e4, 8
Ambulatory care, 50, 80
American Academy for Advancement of Sciences, 58–59
American Academy of Family Physicians, 53
American College of Human Genetics, 19
American College of Medical Genetics, 4, 61
American Nurses Association, 21, 49, 51
American Society of Human Genetics, 4, 16, 94
Apolipoprotein e4, 7–8, 82

B

Bipolar affective disorder, 7
Brain tumors, and Li-Fraumeni syndrome, 34–35

BRCA1. *See* Breast cancer

Breast cancer, 8, 17, 21, 24, 55, 82–83, 87
    early onset, family pedigree example, 36
    inherited susceptibility, 9, 35, 92
    link to Li-Fraumeni syndrome, 34–35
    mammography, 93
    prophylactic mastectomy, 93
    -related gene BRCA1, 9, 24, 34, 92–94
        consequences of negative test result, 9
        discovery, 7
        risk of ovarian cancer and, 35, 93
        screening, 36

C

California State Department of Health Services, 37
Cancer genetics, cancer risk counseling, 34–36
Chinatown Health Clinic, 27–28, 36, 58
Chromosomes, 63–64, 88
Colon cancer, 8, 24, 82–83
    inherited, 87
Common, complex disorders, 82–83
Community
    hospital-based genetic services, 32